W9-DID-536

ACU—ENERGY
By Patti C. Lloyd

Acu-Energy

Copyright 1982 by Patti C. Lloyd
BiWorld Publishers
P.O.Box 1143, Orem, Utah 84057

First Printing
October 1982

Neither the author nor the publisher, directly or indirectly, dispense medical advice. If you use the information contained herein, without the advice of your physician, you are prescribing for yourself, and the author and publisher assume no responsibility.

ISBN 0-89557-060-2

BiWorld Publishers
P.O. Box 1143
Orem, Utah 84057

Dedicated to Peggy White,
who encouraged me to stay around
positive-thinking people.

TABLE OF CONTENTS

FOREWORD

The contents of this book are the results of three years of research and experimentation. The research took place mostly in my health and beauty salon where all types of people enter.

The suggestions for relief presented here are not cures. They are merely aids to help the body heal itself. The ways that the body can help itself have been learned through the ages, by knowledge passed down from generation to generation, or through basic instinct. The principal means through which the body can help itself are herbs, vitamins, minerals, diet, and beneficial types of exercise. Combined, these regimens give a complete approach to healing.

Patti C. Lloyd
Author

INTRODUCTION

This book is a self-help manual, containing directions and illustrations which will show you exactly where to place your hands on your body while using the energizing machine. It can be used everyday in the privacy of your own home to make you feel steadily better. If you find you have a headache, backache, or other painful area, look it up in alphabetical order. On the same page you will also find the correct herbs, vitamins, minerals and diet to help alleviate your dis-ease.

We are now combining the things man has learned or knew instinctively from the beginning of time: deep breathing, directed thinking, eating and exercising correctly. Only a few seconds now and then throughout the day are all you need from your busy life, and you will note your stress factor decreasing.

A mini-trampoline is the means of recirculating your own energy. Instead of pounding your energy into the pavement, as you do when you are jogging in the street, the rubber mesh acts as a non-conductor and puts it back into your own body.

Acupressure is the use of the ancient Chinese method of acupuncture without the use of needles--only pressure in the points. The technique can be very painful when pressure is applied to already tender or sore places. But if you can stand the pain, it works, because the whole body is interrelated, and pressure in one spot will strengthen tissues in another area.

Instead of using pressure on the acupressure points, the coned fingers are gently placed on the points and your own energy is directed to the spot which needs strengthening through the lymphatic system. Hence, strengthening and pain relief are accomplished without adding more pain.

The lymphatic system is an involved system which returns fluids from tissues back into circulation. It has no muscles of its own, and the only way to get a flow is to exercise. The energizing machine enhances this flow. The lymph is collected through the small vessels that merge into the large ones (Black arrows) and is returned (white arrows) to the right side of the heart through veins in the area of the neck. (See p. 205). The lymphatic nodes are along the course of the lymphatic vessles and act as a filter-trap for toxins that are taken into the body through eating and breathing. These nodes stop the spread of infection. That is why it is so important to keep them in good working condition.

Deep breathing is important for relaxation. Breathe in through the nose and out through the mouth. Try to fill your lungs as full as possible with clean air. It the air is polluted, or if someone smokes in your home, it would be wise to have some sort of filter system close to your energizing machine. We like the ion machines.

Directed thinking is important throughout this book. You will find phrases to repeat to get you thinking along positive lines. This is a way of controlling your emotions, which are connected with various ailments. I have chosen phrases which will strengthen specific glands through the control of the emotion involved. The bible is used for many of these phrases, because my research has shown it to be the greatest reference for human emotional control, and most people have on the they can use. As you say these phrases over and over, you do it in rhythm of the bounce of the enrgizing machine. Soon your mind is focused on that, and all negativity is gone. Then healing can take place.

Time element is imperative when beginning to work with the nergizing machine. It is very important to spend only a small amount of time, especially if you are very ill: only 15 to 30 seconds on one acupressure point. It is much better to be on the machine for 30 seconds many times a day than 15 minutes all at once.

GLOSSARY

Coning fingers — Drawing all five fingers close together in a point, fingers only slightly bent.

Deep-breathing — Breath in through the nose and out through the mouth.

Directed thinking — Keeping the mind only on the area to be strengthened.

Energizing — Using a mini trampoline or rebounding machine. The mini trampoline to use for this therapy is constructed in the following manner. All metal including springs, frames and hand rails must be enclosed in a rubber-like substance so that it can remain strictly a non-conductor. If there is metal exposed it will leach the electrical potential of the generating process. The metal legs must also have rubber feet. The rubberized mesh must be taut for best results. The best construction is in the following illustrations, and is very important because I have found that exposed metal will short circuit and you will become very weak. The jogging machines with metal exposed are all right for exercising but not for health therapy!

Flat hand technique — use very light hand pressure moving toward lymph node.

Generate — Keep both feet flat on the mini trampoline and bounce slowly up and down.

Lymph nodes — located along the course of the lymphatic vessels (places about the size of your finger tip), they act like a filter trap for toxins taken into your body.

Partner power — Using another friend to place their fingers on acu-pressure points which are either uncomfortable for you to reach or if you are unable to stand on the energizing machine, your friend can lay you on it, or put your feet on it while you sit in your easy chair and he does the generating. Either you or your friend can place fingers on the acupressure points.

Pin Point — Place coned fingers on the exact point of pain with one hand and the coned fingers of other hand on lymphatic node.

Squeezing — Motion like kneading bread, using a pressing action with fingers and palms. Place hands on hips, fingers in back, thumbs in front.

Stroking — Place coned fingers of one hand on lymphatic node. With coned fingers of other hand use long, steady motions over the area you are working on.

TESTIMONIALS

Experience is the best teacher, so I am going to share some things that have happened to my friends and me while using the programs featured in this book.

Let's start with me. I had more problems than a Ubangi with chapped lips! I was never a strong child to begin with. At age 7 I had Rheumatic Fever and ever since I can remember I've been plagued with migraine headaches which would keep me in bed for a couple of days. I was as nervous as a cat and tired most of the time. My folks called me their "million dollar baby" because of all the doctors, clinics and hospitals I visited without much noticeable relief. My teenage years were blessed with 500% acne, and very slow development thus more specialists. Marriage brought miscarriages, shattered nerves and more doctors. Then I had a chance to teach in Belgium, and while over there I noticed I wasn't sick: in fact I felt great. I was eating like the Belgians--fresh vegetables, whole grain breads, and hardly any meat. I got pregnant and had a beautiful, healthy baby. I came back to the United States and started getting sick again, and had more miscarriages. So I went back to eating like a Belgian, with a good natural vitamin program, visits to the chiropractor, and the discovery of the wonderful energizing machine. I still go to the doctor for yearly checkups, but I feel so good when I maintain my program that I don't really need their services anymore.

Karen Draper, Spring Lake, Michigan

My sinuses would just kill me. I would be in bed for days with a sinus headache and just ache all over. With the help of the energizing machine and herbs, I've cut my sick days almost to nothing. I work on the energizing machine religiously, and it has not only resulted in my feeling great, but I also look great because my body is in such great tone.

Wendy Schweifler, Grand Haven, Michigan

Although I am only twelve years old, I have always had a weight problem. I like to watch TV, but now instead of just sitting, I work on the energizing machine. The last pair of jeans I bought were slims, and that makes me feel terrific!

LLoyd Johnson, North Hollywood, California

I've had a history of heart disease for years. Generating on the energizing machine has stregthened my heart to the extent that when I had an angiogram taken, they found I was growing new veins and arteries around the heart damage. In other words, I was growing my own by-pass...beats surgery any day.

Gladys Johnsen, Sylmar, California

I have suffered from arthritis for years. This new method of using the energizing machine has given me relief. I must use the herbs and energizing machine throughout the day, but it is certainly worth a few extra minutes.

SECTION ONE
Health Dictionary

ABDOMINAL PAIN

Herbal Combinations

I   Capsicum, Valerian Root, Wild Lettuce.

4-A   Alfalfa, Comfrey, Horsetail, Irish Moss, Lobelia, Oat Straw.

4-B   Horsetail, Comfrey, Oatstraw, Lobelia.

14   Hops, Scullcap, Valerian Root.

Vitamins

C--large doses.

Minerals

Calcium--large doses.

Diet

Juices.

Energizing

Generate; place the coned fingers of one hand on lymphatic node, the other on the following acupressure locations:

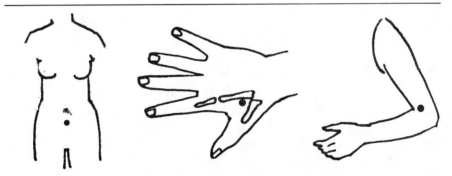

Sit on energizer cross-legged. Generate; place the coned fingers of one hand on lymphatic node, the other on the following acupressure locations:

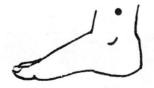

1

ACNE

Herbal Combinations

3-A Barberry, Burdock, Cascara Sagrada, Chapparal, Dandelion, Licorice, Red Clover, Sarsaparilla, Yarrow, Yellow Dock.

3-B Red Clover, Chaparral, Licorice, Peach Bark, Oregon Grape, Stillingia, Cascara Sagrada, Sarsaparilla, Prickly Ash Bark, Burdock, Buckthorn.

Vitamins

A,B,C,E.
Acidophilus.

Diet

Stay away from greasy foods, red meats, acid-forming food and sweets.

Energizing

Generate with partner as often as possible. Cone both hands on upper lymph nodes. Partner cone hands and place on acupressure points pictured:

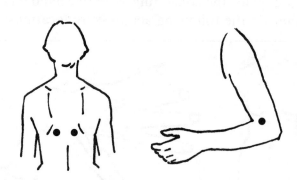

AGE SPOTS

Herbal Combinations

3-A Barberry, Burdock, Cascara Sagrada, Chaparral, Dandelion, Licorice, Red Clover, Sarsaparilla, Yarrow, Yellow Dock.

3-B Red Clover, Chaparral, Licorice, Peach Bark, Oregon Grape, Stillingia, Cascara Sagrada, Sarsaparilla, Prickly Ash Bark, Burdock, Buckthorn.

12-A Cayenne, Ginseng, Gotu Kola.

22-A Angelica, Birch Leaves, Blessed Thistle, Chamomile, Dandelion, Gentian, Golden Rod, Horsetail, Liverwort Leaves. Lobelia, Parsley, Red Beet.

Vitamins

B,E.

Diet

Keep away from synthetic foods and preservatives.

Energizing

Generate; place coned fingers of one hand on lymphatic node, and the other on the following acupressure locations.

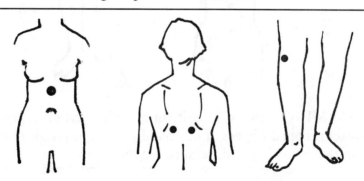

Keeping coned fingers of one hand on the lymphatic node, stroke the area of the liver:

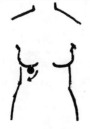

ALCOHOLISM

Herbal Combinations

Help to cleanse the system and take away the taste for alcohol: Capsicum, Golden Seal, Hops, Passion Flower, Saw Palmetto, Scullcap, Valerian Root. (See also Hypoglycemia)

Vitamins

A,B,C,E.

Minerals

Magnesium.

Diet

Stay away from sweets.

Energizing

HANGOVER - Generate, placing coned fingers of one hand on lymphatic node, the other on the following acupressure locations:

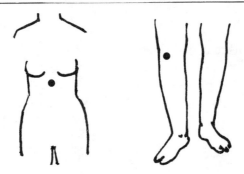

CALMING EFFECT - Sit on energizer cross-legged. Generate; placing coned fingers of one hand on the lymphatic node, the other on the following acupressure location:

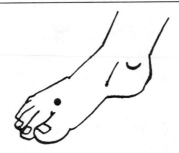

ALLERGIES

Herbal Combinations

4-A Alfalfa, Comfrey, Horsetail, Irish Moss, Lobelia, Oat Straw.

4-B Horsetail, Comfrey, Oatstraw, Lobelia.

10-A Black Cohosh, Blessed Thistle, Pleurisy Root, Scullcap.

10-B Brigham Tea, Marshmallow, Golden Seal Root, Chaparral, Burdock, Parsley, Capsicum, Lobelia.

21-A Comfrey, Lobelia, Marshmallow, Mullein, Slippery Elm.

21-B Marshmallow, Mullein, Comfrey, Lobelia, Chickweed.
Bee Pollen

Vitamins

A,C,E, Pantothenic Acid.

When starting, build up with Alfalfa and Calcium. High doses will not hurt you when you are using the natural form in an herbal base.

Diet

Keep track of what you eat. When you have a reaction, check back on what you've eaten. Keep away from what makes you sick!

Energizing

Generate; placing coned fingers of one hand on the lymphatic node, and the other on the following acupressure locations:

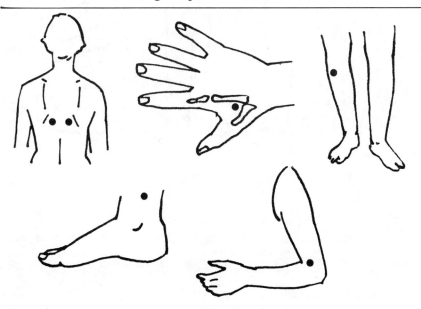

ANEMIA

Herbal Combinations

3-A Barberry, Burdock, Cascara Sagrada, Chaparral, Dandelion, Licorice, Red Clover, Sarsaparilla, Yarrow, Yellow Dock.

3-B Red Clover, Chaparral, Licorice, Peach Bark, Oregon Grape, Stillingia, Cascara Sagrada, Sarsaparilla, Prickly Ash Bark, Burdock, Buckthorn.

19-A Alfalfa, Dandelion, Kelp.

19-B Yellow Dock, Red Beet, Nettle, Burdock, Strawberry Leaves, Mullein, Lobelia.

Vitamins

B,C,E, PABA.

Minerals

Iron.

Diet

Liver (if animals are not raised chemically). Dark green vegetables.

Energizing

Generate; placing coned fingers of one hand on lymphatic node, the other on the following acupressure locations:

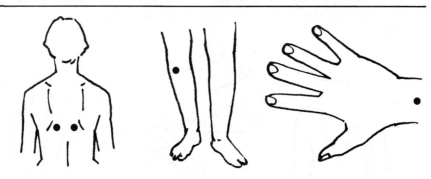

ANXIETY

Herbal Combinations

4-A Alfalfa, Comfrey, Horsetail, Irish Moss, Lobelia, Oatstraw.

4-B Horsetail, Comfrey, Oatstraw, Lobelia,

6-A Black Cohosh, Capsicum, Ginger, Hops, Mistletoe, St. Johnswort, Valerian, Wood Betony.
Horsetail, Comfrey, Oatstraw, Lobelia.

6-B Black Cohosh, Capsicum, Hops, Mistletoe, Lobelia, Scullcap, Wood Betony, Lady's Slipper, Valerian.

Vitamins

B-High doses; this will give you a big appetite, so take the herb Fennel to curb the appetite.

Minerals

Calcium, Iodine, Magnesium.

Diet

Cut down on sugar, acids, coffee, tea (you *can* drink herb teas), and smoking.

Energizing

Generate; placing coned fingers of one hand on lymphactic node, and the other on the following acupressure locations:

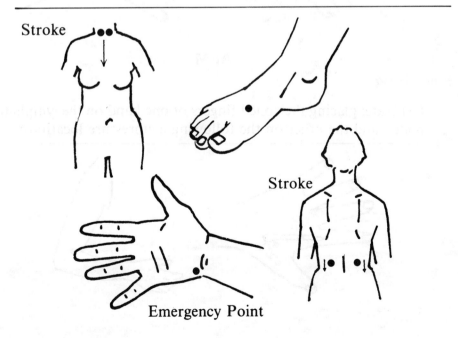

Stroke

Stroke

Emergency Point

APPETITE

Herbal Combinations

To *Increase* appetite: Fennel, Wild Yam, Peppermint, Ginger, Papaya, Spearmint, Catnip, Lobelia.

To *decrease* appetite: Chickweed and Fennel.

Vitamins

Increase: Vitamin B.

Diet

Eat small amounts more often. Stop eating before you get a "stuffed" feeling.

Energizing

Generate; placing the coned fingers of one hand on lymphatic node, and the other in the following acupressure locations:

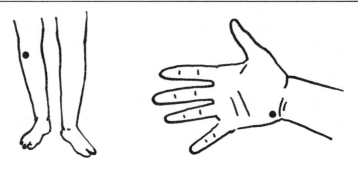

ARM

Energizing

Generate; placing the coned fingers of one hand on the lymphatic node , and the other on the following acupressure locations:

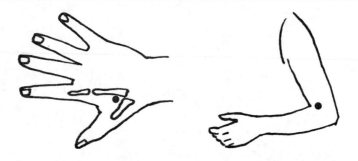

ARTERIOSCLEROSIS

Herbal Combinations

4-A Alfalfa, Comfrey, Horsetail, Irish Moss, Lobelia, Oatstraw.

4-B Horsetail, Comfrey, Oatstraw, Lobelia.

12- Capsicum, Parsley, Ginger, Garlic, Ginseng, Golden Seal Root.

13- Capsicum, Garlic, Hawthorne.

Capsicum and Garlic.

Vitamins

A,B,C,E.

Minerals

Calcium and Magnesium.

Diet

Stay away from fatty foods and salt.

Energizing

Generate; placing coned fingers of one hand on lymphatic node, and the other on the following acupressure locations:

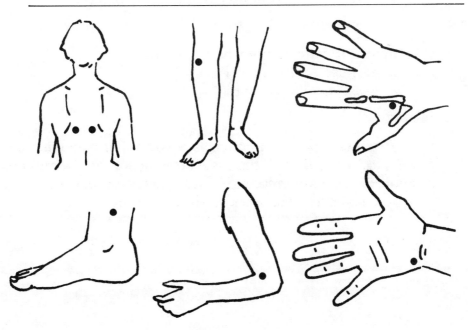

ARTHRITIS

Herbal Combinations

1- Capsicum, Valerian Root, Wild Lettuce.

2- Alfalfa, Black Cohosh, Bromalain Powder, Burdock Root, Capsicum, Centaury, Chaparral, Comfrey, Lobelia, Yarrow, Yucca.
(Add more Alfalfa and Yucca if necessary).

4-A Alfalfa, Comfrey, Horsetail, Irish Moss, Lobelia, Oat Straw.

4-B Horsetail, Comfrey, Oat Straw, Lobelia.

6-A Black Cohosh, Capsicum, Ginger, Hops, Mistletoe, St. Johnswort, Valerian, Wood Betony.

6-B Black Cohosh, Capsicum, Hops, Mistletoe, Lobelia, Scullcap, Wood Betony, Lady's Slipper, Valerian.

Vitamins

A and D before going to bed, or one hour before breakfast in the morning. B,C, and E at another time during the day.

Minerals

Calcium, Potassium and ½ teaspoon mineral water.

Diet

No potatoes or starches-use whole grain rice.
No red meat-use poultry and fish.
No sweets-use many vegetables.

Energizing

Use energizing apparatus as often as possible. For pain relief see: *Hand, Leg, Neck, Back.* If there is acute pain in a specific area not mentioned, generate; placing coned fingers of one hand on lymphatic node, and the other on the area of pain.

ASTHMA

Herbal Combinations

10-A Black Cohosh, Blessed Thistle, Pleurisy Root, Scullcap.

10-B Brigham Tea, Marshmallow, Golden Seal Root, Chaparral, Burdock, Parsley, Capsicum, Lobelia.

21-A Comfrey, Lobelia, Marshmallow, Mullein, Slippery Elm.

21-B Marshmallow, Mullein, Comfrey, Lobelia, Chickweed.

Bee Pollen.

Emergency: Tincture of Lobelia.

Vitamins

A,B, High quantities of Pantothenic Acid.

Minerals

Calcium.

Diet

Low in dairy products. Use honey instead of sugar. (See also *Allergies.*)

Energizing

Place coned fingers and flat hands on lymphatic nodes and chest area with both hands. Generate as long and as often as possible.

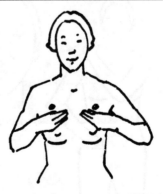

Continue generating; placing coned fingers of one hand on lymphatic node, and the other on the following acupressure locations:

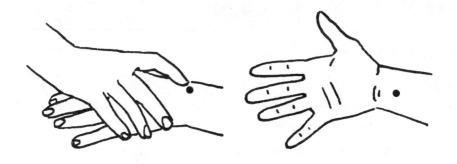

BACK

Herbal Combinations

A-1 Alfalfa, Comfrey, Horsetail, Irish Moss, Lobelia, Oat Straw.

A-2 Horsetail, Comfrey, Oat Straw, Lobelia.

(Add more Alfalfa if necessary).

Minerals

Calcium (vegetable).

Energizing

Generate; placing coned fingers of one hand on lymphatic node, and the other on the following acupressure locations:

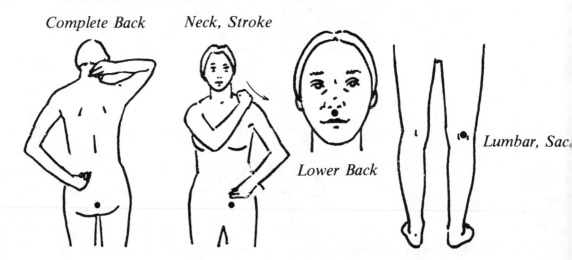

Complete Back   *Neck, Stroke*

Lower Back

Lumbar, Sac.

BAD BREATH

Herbal Combinations

20-A Barberry, Buckthorn, Cascara Sagrada, Capsicum, Couch Grass, Ginger, Licorice, Lobelia, Red Clover.

20-B Cascara Sagrada, Barberry Bark, Capsicum, Ginger, Lobelia, Red Raspberry, Golden Seal Root, Fennel, Turkey Rhubarb Root.
   Clean teeth and gums with Myrrh.

Vitamins

C.
Liquid Chlorophyll.

Diet

Stay off red meat for awhile and eat green vegetables freely.

Energizing

Generate; placing coned fingers of one hand on lymphatic node, and the other on the following acupressure locations:

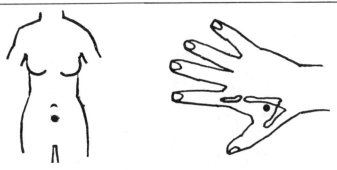

Keeping coned fingers of one hand on lymphatic node, *stroke* the area of the colon: *Stroke* upwards on the right side, sideways from right to left across the navel, then downwards on the left side. Continue generating and place your flat hand on your abdomen.

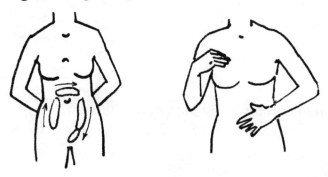

BALDNESS

Herbal Combinations

41-   Dulse, Horsetail, Sage, Rosemary

Jojoba Oil. Massage into the scalp as often as possible with a small, circular motion. Head down to knees for better circulation. Shampoo with mild herbal shampoo.

Vitamins

B,C,E.

Diet

Stay away from chemical food and preservatives.

Energizing

Generate; placing coned fingers of one hand on lymphatic node, and the other on the following acupressure locations:

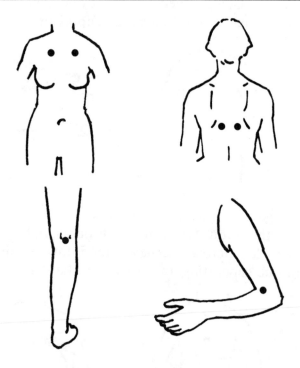

Continue generating, and advance into a bounce if possible, with both flat hands on balding area. Do not have hands touching each other.

BED WETTING

Herbal Combinations

6-A Black Cohosh, Capsicum, Ginger, Hops, Mistletoe, St. Johnswort, Valerian, Wood Betony.

6-B Black Cohosh, Capsicum, Hops, Mistletoe, Lobelia, Scullcap, Wood Betony, Lady's Slipper, Valerian.

18-A Chamomile, Dandelion, Juniper, Parsley, Uva Ursi.

18-B Juniper Berries, Parsley, Uva Ursi, Marshmallow, Lobelia, Ginger, Golden Seal Root.

18-C Juniper Berries, Uva Ursi, Parsley, Black Cohosh, Marshmallow, White Pond Lily, Ginger, Lobelia, Gravel Root, Cornsilk.

One cup Parsley Tea on hour before bedtime.

Vitamins

A.

Minerals

Magnesium.

Diet

Low Salt.

Energizing

Generate; placing coned fingers of one hand on lymphatic node, and the other on the following acupressure locations:

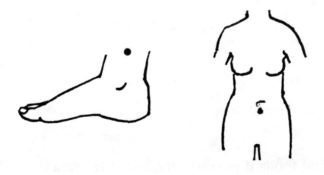

BEE STINGS
(See also: *Bites*).

Herbal Combinations

4-A Alfalfa, Comfrey, Horsetail, Irish Moss, Lobelia, Oat Straw.

4-B Horsetail, Comfrey, Oat Straw, Lobelia.

10-A Black Cohosh, Blessed Thistle, Pleurisy Root, Scullcap.

10-B Brigham Tea, Marshmallow, Golden Seal Root, Chaparral, Burdock, Parsley, Capsicum, Lobelia.

Honey pulls stinger out, and helps neutralize poison. Apply ice until swelling goes down. Apply Redmond Clay.

Vitamins

C.

Minerals

Calcium, Magnesium.

Energizing

DANGER: Do NOT use machine if allergic. Otherwise: Generate; place coned fingers of one hand on lymphatic node, and the other on pin point of pain.

BIRTH DEFECTS
(prevention of).

Herbal Combinations

19-A Alfalfa, Dandelion, Kelp.

Raspberry.

Vitamins

A,E.

Minerals

Manganese, Phosphorus.

Energizing

Eat natural foods if possible--the less processing the better--raw preferred. Low on red meats, sugar and salt.
(See *Pregnancy*).

BITES

(All insects, including poisonous. See also: *Bee Stings* and *Lice*).

Herbal Combinations

4-A Alfalfa, Comfrey, Horsetail, Iris Moss, Lobelia, Oat Straw.

4-B Horsetail, Comfrey, Oat Straw, Lobelia.

Juniper Berry for itching--internal and external.

Liquid Chlorophyll.

Vitamins

C, B complex all year round helps prevent insects from biting in the first place.

Minerals

Calcium, Magnesium.

Diet

Eat as many Dark green vegetables as you can get down. Smaller amounts of meats and sweets.

Energizing

(See: *Nerves* and *Itching*).

BLADDER

Bladder (See also: *Kidneys, Urination*).

Herbal Combinations

18-A Chamomile, Dandelion, Juniper, Parsley, Uva-Ursi.

18-B Juniper Berries, Parsley, Uva-Ursi, Marshmallow, Lobelia, Ginger, Golden Seal Root.

18-C Juniper Berries, Uva-Ursi, Parsley, Black Cohosh, Marshmallow, White Pond Lily, Ginger, Lobelia, Gravel Root, Cornsilk.

Constant seepage--Peach Bark.

Hemorrhage--1 oz. Marshmallow in 1 pt. milk, simmer slowly. Then take ½ cup every ½ hour.

Energizing

Generate; placing coned fingers of one hand on lymphatic node, the other on the following acupressure locations and think about being very patient.

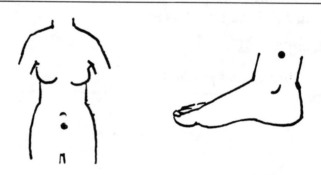

BLOOD PRESSURE

High Blood Pressure, Hypertension

Herbal Combinations

13-A Capsicum, Garlic, Hawthorne.

Capsicum and Garlic.

Vitamins

B and C.

Minerals

Magnesium, Potassium.

Diet

(See chart: *Food Best for Human Consumption*).

Energizing

Generate; placing the coned fingers of one hand on the lymphatic node, the other on the following acupressure locations:

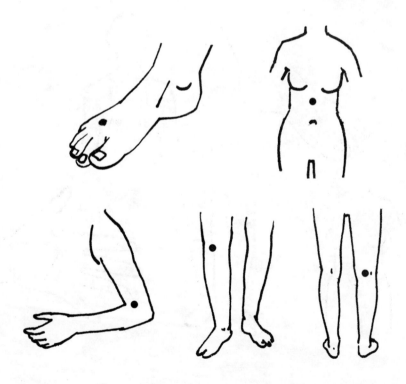

BLOOD PRESSURE
Low Blood Pressure, Hypotension

Herbal Combinations

13-B Capsicum, Parsley, Ginger, Garlic, Ginseng, Golden Seal Root.
Dandelion.

Vitamins

B, C, E.

Minerals

Calcium, Magnesium.

Diet

(See chart: *Food Best for Human Consumption*).

Energizing

Generate; placing coned fingers of one hand on lymphatic node and the other on the following acupressure locations:

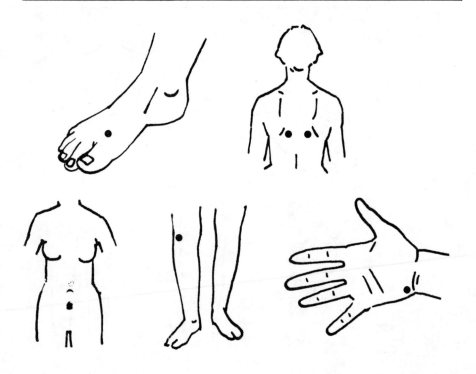

BLOOD PURIFIER

Herbal Combinations

3-A Barberry, Burdock, Cascara Sagrada, Chaparral, Dandelion, Licorice, Red Clover, Sarsaparilla, Yarrow, Yellow Dock.

3-B Red Clover, Chaparral, Licorice, Peach Bark, Oregon Grape, Stillingia, Cascara Sagrada, Sarsaparilla, Prickly Ash Bark, Burdock, Buchthorn.

Diet

(See: *Seven Day Cleanse*). When you resume eating, stay away from chemical foods and preservatives.

Energizing

Generate; placing coned fingers of one hand on lymphatic node, and the other on the following acupressure locations:

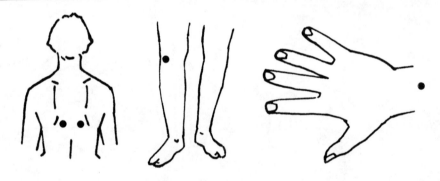

BOILS

Herbal Combinations

Make Compress:

24-B   Comfrey, White Oak Bark, Mullein, Black Walnut, Marshmallow, Gravel Root, Wormwood, Lobelia, Scullcap.

Poultice: 3 parts Mullein to 1 part Lobelia.

Vitamins

B complex.

Diet

(See chart: *Food Best for Human Consumption*).

Energizing

Generate; placing the coned fingers of one hand on lymphatic node, and the other on the following acupressure locations:

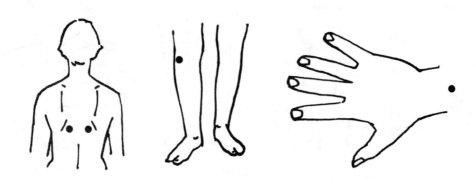

BONES

Herbal Combinations

4-A Alfalfa, Comfrey, Horsetail, Irish Moss, Lobelia, Oat Straw.

4-B Horsetail, Comfrey, Oat Straw, Lobelia.

24-A Aloe Vera, Comfrey, Golden Seal, Slippery Elm.

Vitamins

E.

Minerals

Calcium, Phosphorus.

Diet

Soy bean protein powder at one meal per day.

Energizing

(See also specific bones).
Generate; placing the coned fingers of on hand on lymphatic node, the other on the following acupressure location:

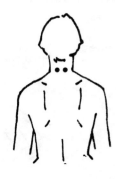

BRAIN
Brain and Psychic Disorders

Herbal Combinations

19-A Alfalfa, Dandelion, Kelp.

19-B Yellow Dock, Red Beet, Nettle, Burdock, Strawberry Leaves, Mullein, Lobelia.

Gota Kola

Vitamins

B complex, and C in large amounts, E, A, and D (Cod liver oil).

Minerals

Iron, Calcium, Magnesium.

Diet

Large amount of Soybean protein powder; eliminate all sugar; reduce all salt; eat liver, eggs, and 100% whole grain bread often.

Energizing

May have to generate with partner at first. When able to generate alone, place coned fingers of one hand on lymphatic node, and the other on the following acupressure locations:

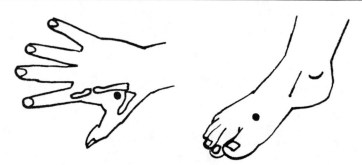

BREASTS

Breasts (See also: *Mastitis*).

Herbal Combinations

To *Increase* size:

Saw Palmetto.
Red Raspberry.

Vitamins

A,C,E.

Diet

Soybean protein powder at every meal.

Energizing

This is the most important aspect. Generate; placing coned fingers of one hand on lymphatic node, and the other on the following acupressure locations:

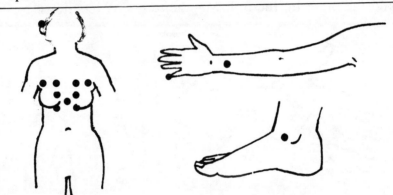

Herbal Combinations

To *Decrease* size:

8-A   Blessed Thistle, Capsicum, Ginger, Golden Seal, Gravel Root, Lobelia, Marshmallow, Parsley, Raspberry.

Dong Quai.

Use cold compresses or even ice packs up to 3 times per day.

Energizing

Gernerate; placing coned fingers and flat hands on lymphatic nodes and chest area with both hands. Generate as long and as often as possible

BREATHING DIFFICULTY
(See also: *Nose, Asthma*)

Herbal Combinations

13-A Capsicum, Garlic, Hawthorne.

21-A Comfrey, Lobelia, Marshmallow, Mullein, Slippery Elm.

Vitamins

Good natural multiple vitamin, E and lecithin.

Minerals

Calcium and Magnesium.

Diet

See: *Food Best for Human Consumption.*

Energizing

Generate; placing coned fingers of one hand on lymphatic node, and the other on the following acupressure locations:

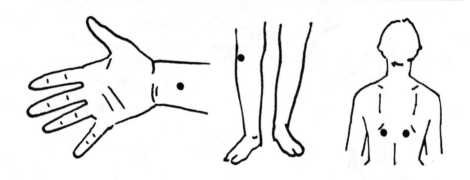

BRONCHITIS

Herbal Combinations

5-A   Capsicum, Chamomile, Golden Seal, Lemon Grass, Myrrh, Peppermint, Rose Hips, Sage, Slippery Elm, Yarrow.

5-B   Garlic, Rosehips, Rosemary, Parsley, Watercress.

10-A   Black Cohosh, Blessed Thistle, Pleurisy Root, Scullcap.

10-B   Brigham Tea, Marshmallow, Golden Seal Root, Chaparral, Burdock, Parsley, Capsicum, Lobelia.

21-A   Comfrey, Lobelia, Marshmallow, Mullein, Slippery Elm.

21-B   Marshmallow, Mullein, Comfrey, Lobelia, Chickweed.

Vitamins

A,C,E.

Diet

Stay away from dairy products.

Energizing

Generate; placing coned fingers of one hand on lymphatic node, and the other on the following acupressure locations:

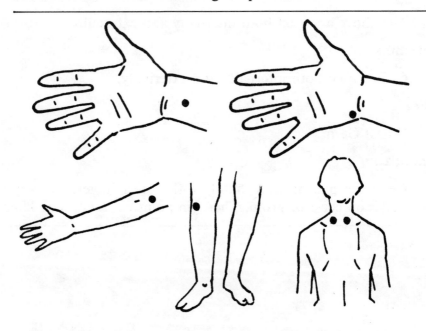

BRUISES

(See also: *Inflammation*).

Herbal Combinations

Comfrey, Fenugreek, White Oah Bark.
All herbs above are beneficial when taken internally, or when used as a poultice.

Vitamins

C,E.

Minerals

Calcium.

Energizing

DANGER, do not use the machine if there is a hard knot in the area of the bruise.

BURNS

Herbal Combinations

24-A   Aloe Vera, Comfrey, Golden Seal, Slippery Elm.

Aloe Vera.

The above are used both internally and externally.

Vitamins

C. E is used both internally and externally.

Diet

Wheat Germ.

Energizing

Generate; placing both hands with coned fingers on lymphatic nodes on chest or groin. Then pin point pain with one hand.

BURSITIS

(See also: *Arthritis, Rheumatism*).

Herbal Combinations

1- Capsicum, Valerian Root, Wild Lettuce.

2- Alfalfa, Black Cohosh, Bromalain Powder, Burdock Root, Capsicum, Centaury, Chaparral, Comfrey, Lobelia, Yarrow, Yucca.

4-A Alfalfa, Comfrey, Horsetail, Irish Moss, Lobelia, Oat Straw.

4-B Horsetail, Comfrey, Oat Straw, Lobelia.

Poultice--Mullein.

Vitamins

C.

Minerals

Calcium.

Energizing

Generate; placing coned fingers of one hand on lymphatic node, and the other on the following acupressure locations:

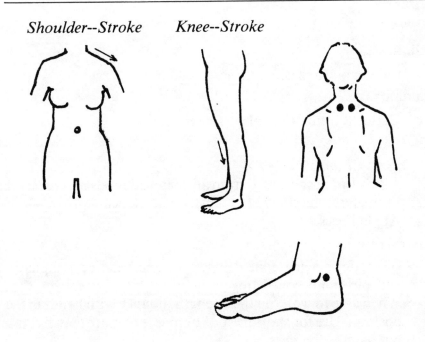

Shoulder--Stroke　　*Knee--Stroke*

CANCER
(See also: *Tumors* and *Cleansing*).

Herbal Combinations

3-A Barberry, Burdock, Cascara Sagrada, Chaparral, Dandelion, Licorice, Red Clover, Sarsaparilla, Yarrow, Yellow Dock.

3-B Red Clover, Chaparral, Licorice, Peach Bark, Oregon Grape, Stillingia, Cascara Sagrada, Sarsaparilla, Prickly Ash Bark, Burdock, Buckthorn.

28-A Barberry, Black Walnut, Catnip, Chickweed, Comfrey, Cyani Flowers, Dandelion, Echinacea, Fenugreek, Gentian, Golden Seal, Irish Moss, Mandrake, Myrrh Gum, Pink Root, Safflowers, St. Johnswort, Yellow Dock.

28-B Cascara Sagrada, Comfrey, Culver's Root, Mandrake, Mullein, Pumpkin Seeds, Slippery Elm, Violet Leaves, Witch Hazel.

Drink as much Red Clover Tea as possible.

Daily--Six Red Clover, six combination #28 above (Barberry, Black Walnut, ...etcetera), six Chaparral, six Ginger, and ½ t. mineral water.

Vitamins
A,B,C,E.

Minerals
Calcium, Magnesium, Zinc.

Enemas
Coffee, Catnip. (See also: *Enemas*).

Diet
(See: *Cleansing*).
After cleanse stay away from all chemical foods and preservatives. Drink large amounts of natural, unsweetened Apricot, Grape, and Apple juices.

Energizing
Generate; placing coned fingers of one hand on lymphatic node and pin point coned fingers of other hand where the cancer is. When able to work up the strength, bounce with hands in the same position. Use for short periods of time, not more than five minutes, but as often as possible.

CATARACTS

Herbal Combinations

7-B   Bayberry, Eyebright, Golden Seal, Capsicim.

Take internally and also use as an eyewash. One capsule of the above combination in ¼ c. boiling, distilled water, straind through cotton balls. Use as often as possible--five or six times per day. If solution is too strong, dilute it until your eyes can stand it.

Vitamins

A,B.

Minerals

Calcium.

Diet

Lots of carrots and parsley, juiced if possible.

Energizing

Rub palms of hands together forcefully until you feel heat. Generate; holding palms over eyes.
Breathe Correctly.

CHICKEN POX
(See also: *Contagious Diseases*).

Herbal Combinations

Burdock, Golden Seal, Yellow Dock.

Bathe body with the above herbs to relieve soreness.

Vitamins

C--100 mg. every hour will alleviate itching problems.

Diet

Liquids and juices (not tomato or orange).

Energizing

Generate; placing both hands with coned fingers on lymphatic nodes.

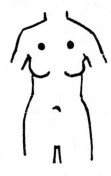

CHOLERA

Herbal Combinations

Valerian Root, Ginger, Peppermint, Cloves, Columba, White Poplar, Slippery Elm, Uva-Ursi, Red Raspberry, Red Clove, and Wild Yam.

Fever

Combine 5 oz. Purple Loosestrife, 1 oz. Ginger, crushed with 3 pints distilled water. Simmer mixture until 1½ pints remain. Give small amount every half hour.

OR

Combine 4 tsp. Black Pepper, 3-4 tbsp. sea salt. ½ cup of warm water and ½ cup Apple Cider Vinegar. Give 1 tbsp. 3 times daily.

Enemas

Bayberry and Catnip (see also: *Enemas*).
Bistort--Make tea and inject in rectum.

Diet

Rice water, leaves of peach, raspberry and sunflowers.

Energizing

Generate; placing coned fingers of one hand on lymphatic node, and the other on the following acupressure locations:

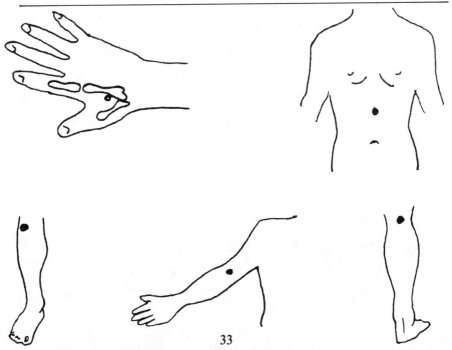

CIRCULATION

Herbal Combinations

13-A Capsicum, Garlic, Hawthorn.

13-B Capsicum, Parsley, Ginger, Garlic, Ginseng, Golden Seal Root.

Capsicum increases pulse rate.
Black Cohosh decreases pulse rate.

Vitamins

C, E, Lecithin.

Minerals

Calcium.

Diet

See: *Food Best for Human Consumption.*

Energizing

Jog on machine until heart is beating fast and breathing is heavy, then slow down and generate with coned fingers on lymph nodes until breathing is normal.

COCCYX
(See also: *Back*).

Energizing

Generate; placing the coned fingers of one hand on lymphatic node, and the other on the following acupressure location.

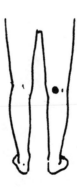

COLDS

(See also: *Cough, Fever, Flu, Mucous*).

Herbal Combinations

4-A Alfalfa, Comfrey, Horsetail, Irish Moss, Lobelia, Oat Straw.

4-B Horsetail, Comfrey, Oat Straw, Lobelia.

5-A Capsicum, Chamomile, Golden Seal, Lemon Grass, Myrrh, Peppermint, Rose Hips, Sage, Slippery Elm, Yarrow.

5-B Garlic, Rose Hips, Rosemary, Parsley, Watercress.

11- Capsicum, Ginger, Golden Seal, Licorice.

Vitamins

A,B,C,E.

Minerals

Calcium.

Diet

See: *Food Best for Human Consumption*

Energizing

Generate; placing coned fingers of one hand on lymphatic node, the other on the following acupressure locations.

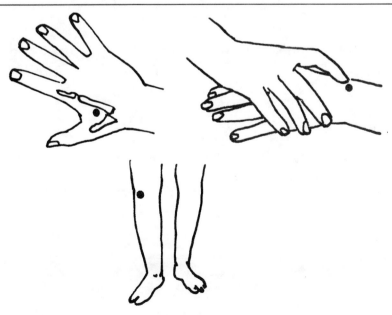

COLD HANDS AND FEET

Herbal Combinations

11- Capsicum, Ginger, Golden Seal, Licorice.

Vitamins

E.

Minerals

Calcium.

Diet

See:*Food Best for Human Consumption.*

Energizing

See: *Circulation.*

COLIC

Herbal Combinations

17- Fennel, Wild Yam, Peppermint, Ginger, Papaya, Spearmint, Catnip, Lobelia.

22-B Barberry Bark, Cramp Bark, Fennel, Ginger, Catnip, Peppermint, Wild Yam.

Make into tea and add honey to taste.

Enemas

Catnip (see: *Enemas*).

Energizing

Generate gently with baby in your arms or place baby on machine and generate with your foot.

COLON

(See: *Colitis, Parasites, Intestines*)

Herbal Combinations

20-A Barberry, Buckthorn, Cascara Sagrada, Capsicum, Couch Grass, Ginger, Licorice, Lobelia, Red Clover.

3-A Cascara Sagrada, Barberry Bark, Capsicum, Ginger, Lobelia, Red Raspberry, Golden Seal Root, Fennel, Turkey Rhubarb Root.

28-A Barberry, Black Walnut, Catnip, Chickweed, Comfrey, Cyani Flowers, Dandelion, Echinacea, Fenugreek, Gentian, Golden Seal, Irish Moss, Mandrake, Myrrh Gum, Pink Root, Safflowers, St. Johnswort, Yellow Dock.

28-B Cascara Sagrada, Comfrey, Culver's Root, Mandrake, Mullein, Pumpkin Seeds, Slippery Elm, Violet Leaves, Witch Hazel.

30-A Capsicum, Golden Seal, Myrrh.

30-B Marshmallow, Slippery Elm, Comfrey, Lobelia, Ginger, Wild Yam.
Fenugreek to lubricate.
Hyssop and Mullein for mucous in the colon.

Vitamins

B,C,E.

Minerals

Calcium, Magnesium, Zinc.

Diet

Steamed Vegetables. (See also: *Colon Therapy Diet*)

Energizing

Generate; placing coned fingers of one hand on lymphatic node, and the other on the following acupressure locations:

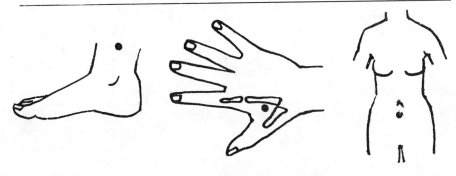

COLITIS

Herbal Combinations

4-A   Alfalfa, Comfrey, Horsetail, Irish Moss, Lobelia, Oat Straw.

4-B   Horsetail, Comfrey, Oat Straw, Lobelia.

20-A   Barberry, Buckthorn, Cascara Sagrada, Capsicum, Couch Grass, Ginger, Licorice, Lobelia, Red Clover.

3-A   Cascara Sagrada, Barberry Bark, Capsicum, Ginger, Lobelia, Red Raspberry, Golden Seal Root, Fennel, Turkey Rhubarb Root,

30-A   Capsicum, Golden Seal, Myrrh.

30B   Marshmallow, Slippery Elm, Comfrey, Lobelia, Ginger, Wild Yam.

Vitamins

B.

Minerals

Calcium, Magnesium.

Diet

low fiber until healed. (Refer to: *Colon Therapy Diet*)

Enemas

White Oak Bark or Slippery Elm. (Also see: *Enemas*).

Energizing

Generate; placing coned fingers of one hand on lymphatic node, and the other on the following acupressure locations:

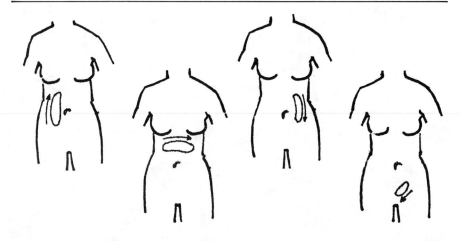

CONSTIPATION
(See also: *Colitis, Colon*).

Herbal Combinations

Cascara Sagrada.

Aloe Vera--1 oz. 4 to 5 times a day.

Diet

High Fiber--raw bran on cereal, or bran muffins are helpful.
Fruit--raw or dried.
Water--at lease 8—8 oz. glasses pure water

Energizing

Generate; placing coned fingers of one hand on lymphatic node, and the other on the following acupressure locations:

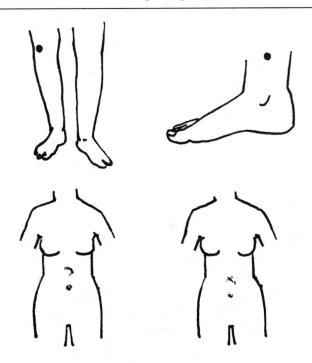

CONTAGIOUS DISEASES

Contagious Diseases (See: *Chicken Pox, Croup, Scarlet Fever, Measles, Mumps, Rhematic Fever, Pink Eye*).

CONVULSIONS

Herbal Combinations

3-A Barberry, Burdock, Cascara Sagrada, Chaparral, Dandelion, Licorice, Red Clover, Sarsaparilla, Yarrow, Yellow Dock.

4-A Alfalfa, Comfrey, Horsetail, Irish Moss, Lobelia, Oat Straw.

6-A Black Cohosh, Capsicum, Ginger, Hops, Mistletoe, St. Johnswort, Valerian, Wood Betony.

14- Hops, Scullcap, Valerian Root.

19-A Alfalfa, Dandelion, Kelp.

29-A Capsicum, Irish Moss, Kelp, Parsley.

Vitamins

A,B,C,D,E.

Minerals

Calcium, Magnesium, Silicone, Zinc.

Diet

Imperative that chemical foods and preservatives are not eaten.

Energizing

Generate; placing coned fingers of one hand on lymphatic node, and the other on the following acupressure locations:

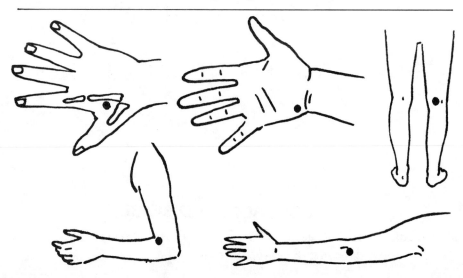

COUGH

Herbal Combinations

21-A Comfrey, Lobelia, Marshmallow, Mullein, Slippery Elm.

21-B Marshmallow, Mullein, Comfrey, Lobelia, Chickweed.

Tincture of Lobelia.
Herbal Punch.
Herbal Cough Syrup.

Vitamins

A.C.

Diet

Keep away from dairy products. (See also: *Food Best for Human Consumption*).

Energizing

Generate; placing coned fingers of one hand on lymphatic node, and the other on the following acupressure locations:

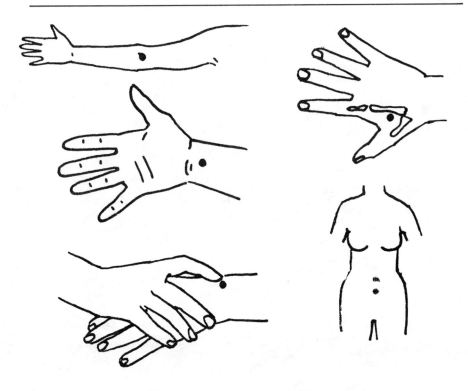

CRAMPS
(Leg, Foot and Writer's Cramp).

Herbal Combinations

4-A Alfalfa, Comfrey, Horsetail, Irish Moss, Lobelia, Oat Straw.

19-B Yellow Dock, Red Beet, Nettle, Burdock, Strawberry Leaves, Mullein, Lobelia.

24-A Aloe Vera, Comfrey, Golden Seal, Slippery Elm.

Vitamins

B,C.

Minerals

Calcium.

Energizing

Generate; placing coned fingers of one hand on lymphatic node, the other on the following acupressure locations:

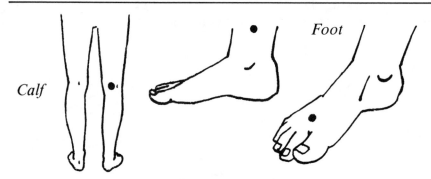

Can also *Stroke* pained area toward nearest lymphatic node.

For Writer's Cramp:

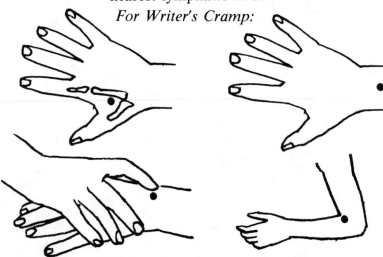

CRAMPS
(Menstral)

Herbal Combinations

1- Cayenne, Valerian Root, Wild Lettuce.

4 A Alfalfa, Comfrey, Horsetail, Irish Moss, Lobelia, Oat Straw.

Red Raspberry Tea.

Energizing

Generate; placing coned fingers of one hand on lymphatic node, and the other on the following acupressure locations:

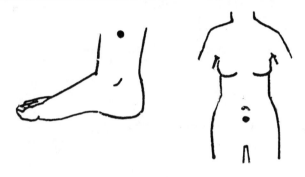

(Stomach)

Herbal Combinations

11- Capsicum, Ginger, Golden Seal, Licorice.

19-A Alfalfa, Dandelion, Kelp.

Minerals

Calcium, Magnesium.

Energizing

Generate; placing the coned fingers of one hand on lymphatic node, and with the other *stroke* the stomach area.

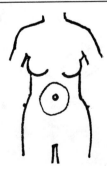

CROUP

Herbal Combinations

20-A Barberry, Buckthorn, Cascara Sagrada, Capsicum, Couch Grass, Ginger, Licorice, Lobelia, Red Clover.

Bayberry--break capsule and blow powder up nostrils.

Tincture of Lobelia--for acute attack.

Ginger Bath--3tbsp. (27 capsules) in a tub of hot water, and put right to bed.

Hot Compress--1 cup cider vinegar and ½ cup salt to 2 quarts hot water. Apply several times daily.

Onion Pack-- Cut onions into small pieces and put into soft cloth. Place on throat and chest.

Enemas

Garlic and Catnip. (See also: *Enemas*).

Diet

Juices and raw vegetables such as Spinach, Parsley, Carrot tops, Beet tops, Comfrey juiced with water and honey to taste. Stay away from sweets, soft drinks, and milk products.

Energizing

Generate with baby in your arms, or lay baby on machine and generate with your foot. If child is big enough, have him generate with both hands with coned fingers on the chest area.

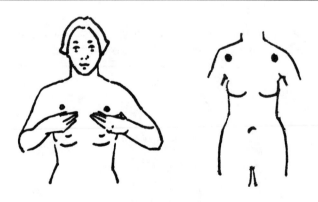

CYSTITIS
(See also: *Bladder* and *Urethra*).

Herbal Combinations

Generate; placing the coned fingers of one hand on lymphatic node, and the other on the following acupressure locations:

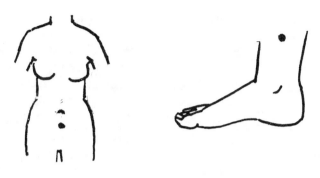

CUTS
(See: *Wounds*).

DANDRUFF

Herbal Combinations

Jojoba--Massage directly onto scalp. Dry scalp after shampooing and do not rinse off. For oily scalp, apply after shampoo. Let stay on for as long as possible, then shampoo off.

Chaparral and Yarrow--Make tea and rinse scalp.

Vitamins

B.

Diet

(See: *Correct Food Combinations*).

Energizing

Generate; placing the coned fingers of one hand on lymphatic node, and the other on the following acupressure location:

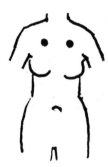

Continue generating; running fingers of both hands through hair, so that all fingers and palms are touching scalp. Repeat,"Every day in every way, I'm getting better and better!" to the rhythm of the bounce.

DEAFNESS
(See also: *Ears*)

Herbal Combinations

37- Extract of Chickweed, Black Cohosh Root, Golden Seal Root, Lobelia, Scullcap, Brigham Tea and Licorice Root.

Drop 6 drops of garlic oil in ear, with 3-6 drops of above combination in ear. Put in soft piece of cotton. Do this for six nights. On the seventh night wash ear with solution of warm apple cider vinegar and distilled water, mix half and half. Use an ear syringe in order to remove all matter from the ear. Continue routine.

Vitamins

C, in large amounts.

Diet

(See: *Food Best for Human Consumption*).

Energizing

Generate; placing the coned fingers of one hand on lymphatic node, and the other on the following acupressure locations:

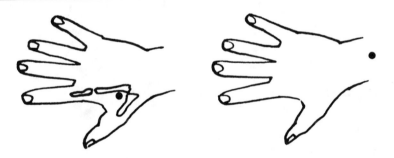

Continue gererating, folding soft part of ear nearest face into ears with coned fingers of both hands. With the nail of the middle finger, tap the nail of the index finger rhythmically. It should have a hollow sound. Then place palms of hands over ears and tap the back of your head rhythmically.

DEPRESSION
(See: Lung).

Herbal Combinations

19-A   Alfalfa, Dandelion, Kelp. (Use large amounts).

Vitamins

B. Large amounts with Fennel to keep appetite controlled.

Diet

No starches or sweets.

Energizing

Generate; placing the coned fingers of one hand on lymphatic node, and the other on the acupressure locations illustrated below. While in this position, try to think cheerful thoughts. Directed thinking is very important here. If you can't think of anything, keep repeating: "I feel healthy, I feel happy, I feel terrific..." to the rhythm of the bounce.

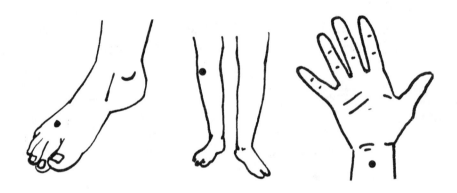

DIAPER RASH
(See also: *Skin Disease*).

Herbal Combinations

Blend Mullein (or Slippery Elm for a paste) with Vitamin E Oil, and apply locally. Garlic Water may also be used.

Enemas

Garlic. (See also: *Enemas*).

Energizing

Generate; hold baby in arms or place baby on machine and generate with your foot.

DIABETES

Herbal Combinations

7 A&B   Bayberry, Capsicum, Eyebright, Golden Seal. (See also: *Eye Wash*).

23-B   Bistort, Blueberry Leaves, Buchu, Calsicum, Comfrey, Dandelion, Garlic, Golden Seal, Juniper Berries, Licorice, Marshmallow, Mullein, Uve-Ursi, Yarrow.

23-C   Juniper Berries, Uva-Ursi, Licorice, Mullein, Capsicum, Golden Seal Root.

Vitamins

A,B,C,E.

Minerals

Potassium.

Diet

Eat small amounts often. Eat as many green vegetables as possible (see: *Correct Food Combinations*). Stay away from sweetes and starches. Eat Blueberries.

Energizing

Generate; place coned fingers of one hand on lymphatic node, the other on the following acupressure locations:

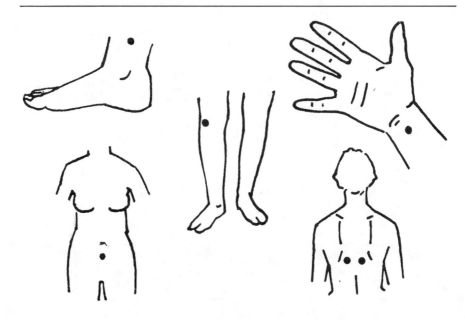

DIARRHEA

Herbal Combinations

Raspberry and Slippery Elm.

½ teasp. nutmeg several times per day.

½ teasp. cloves to 1 quart water for cramping.

Vitamins

B,C.

Minerals

Magnesium.

Enemas

Slippery Elm and Raspberry. (See: *Enemas*).

Diet

Water from cooked rice or oatmeal.
1. Tblsp. Slippery Elm (9 capsules broken) to 1 pint scalded skim milk which has been cooled. Take several times per day.

Energizing

Generate; place coned fingers of one hand on lymphatic node, the other on the following acupressure locations:

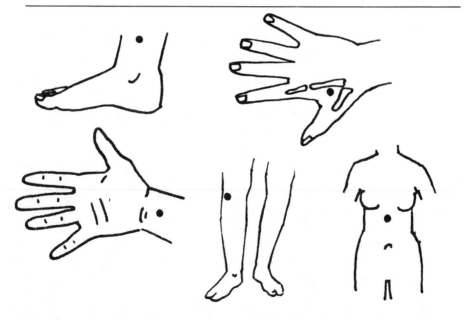

DIGESTION

Herbal Combinations

11-   Capsicum, Ginger, Golden Seal, Licorice.

17-   Fennel, Wild Yam, Peppermint, Ginger, Papaya, Spearmint, Catnip, Lobelia.

30-B Marshmallow, Slippery Elm, Comfrey, Lobelia, Ginger, Wild Yam.

    Aloe Vera.

    Papaya mint and Golden Seal ½ hour before meal.

Vitamins

    B.

Minerals

    Calcium.

Diet

    Low Fat (See also: *Correct Food Combinations*).

Energizing

    Generate; place coned fingers of one hand on lymphatic node, and the other on the following acupressure locations:

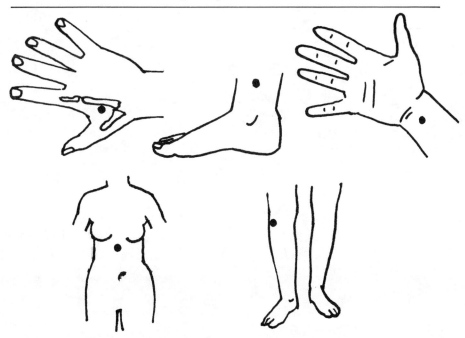

DIURETIC
(See: *Water Retention*).

DIVERTICULITIS
(See: *Colon*).

DIZZINESS

Herbal Combinations

22-A Angelica, Birch Leaves, Blessed Thistle, Chamomile, Dandelion, Gentian, Golden Rod, Horsetail, Liverwort Leaves, Lobelia, Parsley, Red Beet.

Diet

Stay away from chemical foods and preservatives.

Energizing

Generate; place the coned fingers of one hand on lymphatic node, and the other on the following acupressure locations:

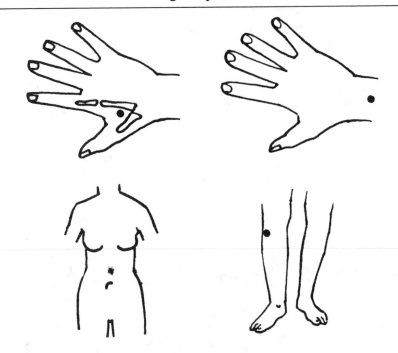

DOUCHE

Herbal Combinations

35- Squawvine, Chickweed, Slippery Elm, Comfrey, Yellow Dock, Golden Seal Root, Mullein, Marshmallow. Use 1 tsp. in 1 pint pure water. Steep and cool.

Fresh Garlic--4-5 crushed cloves to 1 quart of pure water in blender.

Capsicum and Garlic--¼ tsp. od Capsicum and 2-3 crushed Garlic, or open 2 capsules to 1 quart water. Good if you can stand it.

Mineral Water--2 pints to 2 pints pure water.

Marshmallow Tea--5 capsules opened (for irritation).

Bistort Tea for bleeding.

Energizing

See: *Vagina*

DRUG WITHDRAWAL

Herbal Combinations

6-A   Black Cohosh, Capsicum, Ginger, Hops, Mistletoe, St. Johnswort, Valerian, Wood Betony.

6-B   Black Cohosh, Capsicum, Hops, Mistletoe, Lobelia, Scullcap, Wood Betony, Lady's Slipper, Valerian.

12-A   Capsicum, Ginseng, Gotu Kola.

Chamomile, Ginseng, Licorice Root.

Note: *Must take all these herbs for best results.*

Vitamins

B, C, E.

Diet

No sugar or refined starches. (See also: *Correct Food Combinations*).

Energizing

Generate; place coned fingers of one hand on lymphatic node, and the other on the following acupressure location.,

---

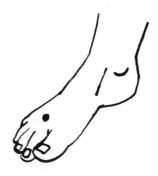

DYSENTARY
(See: *Colon, Diarrhea*).

ECZEMA
(See also: *Skin Disease*).

Herbal Combinations

3-A Barberry, Burdock, Cascara Sagrada, Chaparral, Dandelion, Licorice, Red Clover, Sarsaparilla, Yarrow, Yellow Dock.

4-A Alfalfa, Comfrey, Horsetail, Irish Moss, Lobelia, Oat Straw.

4-B Horsetail, Comfrey, Oat Straw, Lobelia.

6-A Black Cohosh, Cayenne, Ginger, Hops, Mistletoe, St. Johnswort, Valerian, Wood Betony.

20-A Barberry, Buckthorn, Cascara Sagrada, Capsicum, Couch Grass, Ginger, Licorice, Lobelia, Red Clover.

Aloe Vera--Both internally and externally.

Vitamins

A, B, C, Lecithin, PABA.

Minerals

Calcium, Zinc.

Diet

Acidophilus and Yogurt (See also: *Correct Food Combinations*).

Energizing

Generate; place the coned fingers of one hand on lymphatic node, the other on the following acupressure locations:

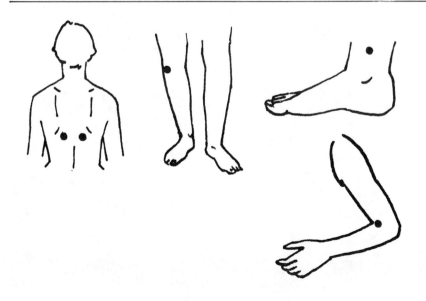

EAR

(See also: *Deafness* and *Meniere's Syndrome*).

Infection or Otitis

Herbal Combinations

5-A Capsicum, Chamomile, Golden Seal, Lemon Grass, Myrrh, Peppermint, Rose Hips, Sage, Slippery Elm, Yarrow.

16-A Capsicum, Echinacea, Myrrh, Yarrow.

16-B Capsicum, Echinacea, Golden Seal, Yarrow.

20-A Barberry, Buckthorn, Cascara Sagrada, Capsicum, Couch Grass, Ginger, Licorice, Lobelia, Red Clover.

37- Extract--Chickweed, Black Cohosh, Golden Seal, Lobelia, Scullcap, Brigham Tea, Licorice (2 drops above extract with 2 drops Garlic Oil for earache). Could also pack ear in ice.

Vitamins

A, C, E.

Minerals

Calcium.

Diet

(See: *Foods Best for Human Consumption*).

Energizing

Generate; place the coned fingers of one hand on lymphatic node, the other on the following acupressure locations:

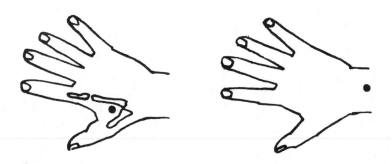

Ear (Continued)

EAR

Ringing in the Ear (Same as Infection or Otitis).

Unsupportive Emotion

Energizing

Generate; place the coned fingers of one hand on lymphatic node, the other *stroking* the following location:

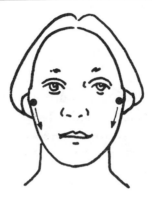

Directed thinking is important when stroking this area. Control your emotions by saying aloud, "God loves me, my husband (wife) loves me, my friends love me, etc., to the rhythm of the bounce. Start with only 30 seconds.

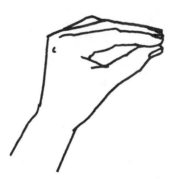

Place the index fingers of each hand on the outside of the ears and fold over the outside flaps of skin which lie next to the opening of the inner ear canal, so that you seal off the ear from the outside. Using tips of second fingers, tap gently on fingernails of index fingers to the rhythm of the bounce.

EDEMA
(Dropsy).

Herbal Combinations

13-A Capsicum, Carlic, Hawthorne.

13-B Capsicum, Parsley, Ginger, Garlic, Ginseng, Golden Seal Root.

Hawthorn Extract--4 droppers full in herbal beverage.

Dandelion.

Diet

Low Salt (See: *Food Best for Human Consumption*).

Energizing

Must start very slowly, use shuffling step, or sit with feet on machine. Generate; place coned fingers of one hand on lymphatic node, the other on the following acupressure location:

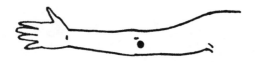

ELBOW PAIN
(Tennis Elbow).

Herbal Combinations

1- Capsicum, Valerian Root, Wild Lettuce.

24-A Aloe Vera, Comfrey, Golden Seal, Slippery Elm - use internally and also make poltice.

Vitamins

B Complex, very high amounts; take Fennel to cut your appetite.

Energizing

Generate; place thew coned fingers of one hand on lymphatic node, the other on the following acupressure locations:

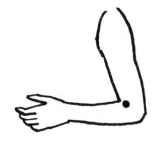

EMPHYSEMA

(See also: *Lungs, Smoking, Breathing Difficulties*).

Herbal Combinations

21-A Comfrey, Lobelia, Marshmallow, Mullein, Slippery Elm.

Comfrey and Fenugreek.

Vitamins

A, B, C, E.

Minerals

Calcium, Magnesium, Zinc.

Diet

Eat whole grains and all vegetables, especially green, leafy ones. Stay away from dairy products and red meat. (See also: *Correct Food Combinations*).

Energizing

Cone thumb and forefingers. Place rest of hand flat on lung area. Generate little by little, until you can stay on for ½ hour.,

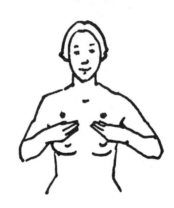

ENDURANCE AND ENERGY
(See also: *Fatigue*).

Herbal Combinations

12-A Capsicum, Ginseng, Gotu Kola.

13-B Capsicum, Parsley, Ginger, Garlic, Ginseng, Golden Seal Root.

19-A Alfalfa, Dandelion, Kelp.

19-B Yellow Dock, Red Beet, Nettle, Burdock, Strawberry Leaves, Mullein, Lobelia.

Vitamins

E.

Diet

High in fruits and vegetables--raw as much as possible.

Energizing

Build up to many high bounces, jogging and kicking. Test your heartbeat, keep working until you sweat and breathe heavily, then slow down and generate until you reach your normal level. Generate; place the coned fingers of one hand on lymphatic node, and the other on the following acupressure locations:

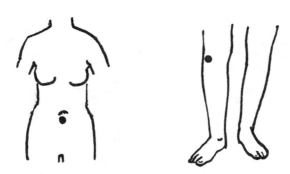

EPILEPSY
(See also: *Convulsions*).

Herbal Combinations

6-A Black Cohosh, Capsicum, Gingers, Hops, Mistletoe, St. Johnswort, Valerian, Wood Betony.

6-B Black Cohosh, Capsicum, Hops, Mistletoe, Lobelia, Scullcap, Wood Betony, Lady's Slipper, Valerian.

Scullcap--Large amounts, religiously.

29-A Capsicum, Irish Moss, Kelp, Parsley.

29-B Parsley, Watercress, Kelp, Irish Moss, Sarsaparilla, Black Walnut, Iceland Moss.

Minerals

Calcium.

Diet

See: *Food Best for Human Consumption.*

Energizing

Generate; place the coned fingers of one hand on lymphatic node, and the other on the following acupressure locations:

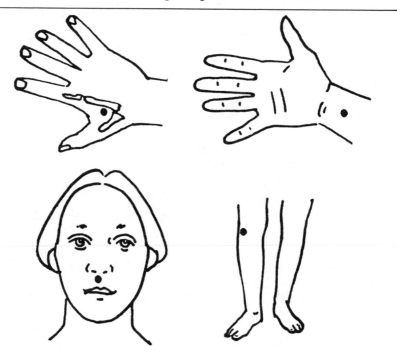

EXHAUSTION
(See: *Fatigue*).

Herbal Combinations

19-A Alfalfa, Dandelion, Kelp. (Large amounts).

Don't push yourself.

Diet

Protein powder along with other food. (See: *Food Best for Human Consumption*). No sugar or refined starches.

Energizing

Generate; place coned fingers on lymphatic area, then strengthen back. Cone fingers on top and bottom of spinal column.

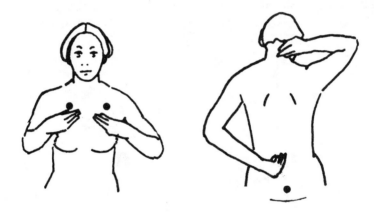

EYES

Herbal Combinations

7 A&B Bayberry, Eyebright, Golden Seal, (Capsicum optional).

Alfalfa, Dandelion, Kelp.

Vitamins

A, B, B2.

Diet

All the carrots and parsley you can eat. (Juice if possible).

Energizing

Rub palms together until warm, place over eyes, generate or bounce on balls of feet. Then generate; place coned fingers of one hand on lymphatic node, the other on the following acupressure locations. Think positively and say aloud, "I will succeed, I will succeed, I will succeed!" to the rhythm of the bounce.

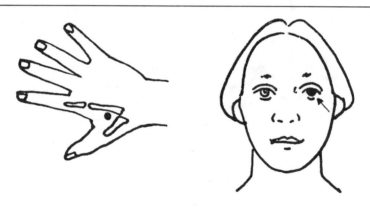

EYE WASH

1 capsule (broken) Herbal Eye Wash (Golden Seal, Bayberry, Eyebright, Red Raspberry Leaves, Capsicum--optional). 1 cup pure water, boiled. Let steep for 20 minutes. Strain through cotton balls in bottom of funnel or tea strainer. Use eye cup or eye dropper. Blink the eye a few times. Let eye rest. Repeat. The eye may sting; if unbearable use more water. Use eye wash at least three times a day. Try to keep eye open while dropping eye wash in. Keep using less and less water as you can stand it. Make new solution every 2 days. Never use the same eyewash potion twice; use fresh solution with each eye.

FACIAL NERVE PARALYSIS

Energizing

Generate; place coned fingers of one hand on lymphatic node, and the other on the following acupressure locations:

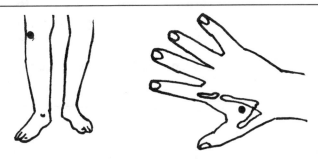

FAINTING

Energizing

Sit with head between knees and feet on machine; generate. For *emergency* place coned fingers of one hand on lymphatic node, and the other on the following acupressure location:

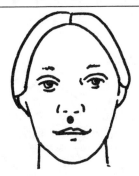

For the following conditions: Sunstroke, Poisoning, Drowning, Choking, Electric Shock, Gas Inhalation, Concussion, Fracture. Generate; place the feet of affected person on machine. Place coned fingers of one hand on lymphatice node, the other on the following acupressure locations:

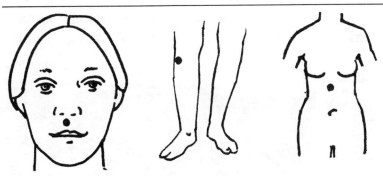

FATIGUE

(See also: *Endurance, Energy*).

Herbal Combinations

12-A Capsicum, Ginseng, Gotu Kola.

13-B Capsicum, Parsley, Ginger, Garlic, Ginseng, Golden Seal Root.

19-A Alfalfa, Dandelion, Kelp.

29-B Parsley, Watercress, Kelp, Irish Moss, Sarsaparilla, Black Walnut, Iceland Moss.

Vitamins

E, Niacin.

Energizing

Mental Fatigue--generate; place coned fingers of one hand on lymphatic node, the other on the following acupressure locations:

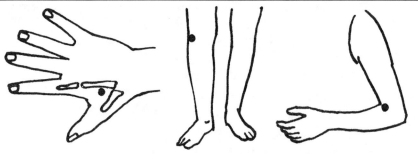

Physical Fatigue--Generate; place coned fingers of one hand on lymphatic node, the other on the following acupressure locations:

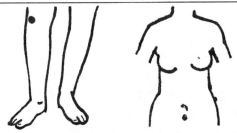

Nerve Fatigue--Generate; place coned fingers of one hand on lymphatic node, and the other on the following acupressure locations:

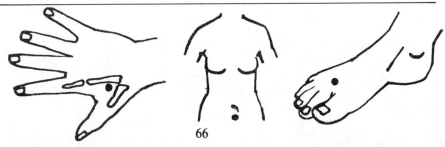

FEET

Herbs

Chamomile--For callouses and corns.

Horsetail--Odor and foot perspiration.

Capsicum--Cold feet.

Energizing

Sit cross-legged on machine. Generate; place coned fingers of one hand on lymphatic node, the other on the following acupressure location. Change hands. Repeat.

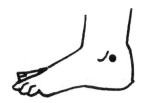

FEMALE PROBLEMS

(See: *Breasts, Frigidity, Hemorrhage, Lactation, Menopause, Menstruation, Miscarriage, Morning Sickness, Child Birth, Pregnancy, Sterility, Uterus*).

FEVER

Herbal Combinations

4-A Alfalfa, Comfrey, Horsetail, Irish Moss, Lobelia, Oat Straw

16-A Capsicum, Echinacea, Myrrh, Yarrow.

16-B Capsicum, Echinacea, Golden Seal, Yarrow.

16-C Plantain, Black Walnut, Golden Seal Root, Bugleweed, Marshmallow, Lobelia.

20-A Barberry, Buckthorn, Cascara Sagrada, Capsicum, Couch Grass, Ginger, Licorice, Lobelia, Red Clover.

Vitamins

C.

Enemas

Catnip--very important (See also: *Enemas*).

Energizing

Generate; place coned fingers of one hand on lymphatic node, the other on the following acupressure locations:

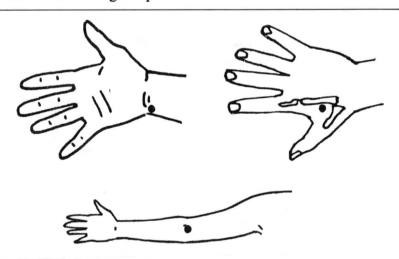

FEVER BLISTERS

Herbal Combinations

3-A   Barberry, Burdock, Cascara Sagrada, Chaparral, Dandelion, Licorice, Red Clover, Sarsaparilla, Yarrow, Yellow Dock.

3-B   Red Clover, Chaparral, Licorice, Poke Root, Peach Bark, Oregon Grape, Stillingia, Cascara Sagrada, Sarsaparilla, Prickly Ash Bark, Burdock, Buckthorn.

30-A   Capsicum, Golden Seal, Myrrh.

30-B   Marshmallow, Slippery Elm, Comfrey, Lobelia, Ginger, Wild Yam.

Aloe Vera--Internally and externally.

White Oak Bark--Internally and externally.

Vitamins

C.

Energizing

Generate; place coned fingers pin pointing fever blister. Place coned fingers of other hand on lymphatic node.

FINGERNAILS

Herbal Combinations

4-A Alfalfa, Comfrey, Horsetail, Irish Moss, Lobelia, Oat Straw.

4-B Horsetail, Comfrey, Oat Straw, Lobelia.

Vitamins

B.

Minerals

Calcium, Potassium.
Length-wise ridges--Iron deficiency--Kelp.
Horizontal lines--iodine deficiency--Kelp.

Diet

(See: *Food Best for Human Consumption*).

Energizing

Generate; pin point coned fingers on each moon of nail. (See also:*Skin Disease*).

FITNESS

Herbal Combinations

38- Ginseng, Ho Shou Wu, Black Walnut Hulls, Licorice, Gentian, Comfrey, Fennel, Bee Pollen, Bayberry, Myrrh, Peppermint, Safflower, Eucalyptus, Lemongrass, Capsicum.

Vitamins

Natural vitamin combination.

Minerals

Natural mineral combination.

Diet

(See: *Correct Food Combination*).

Energizing

The higher the bounce for strength and the higher the jog, the more fit you will become. Build up your time on the machine as well as the frequency with which you use it.

FLU OR INFLUENZA

Herbal Combinations

4-A   Alfalfa, Comfrey, Horsetail, Irish Moss, Lobelia, Oat Straw.

4-B   Horsetail, Comfrey, Oat Straw, Lobelia.

5-A   Capsicum, Chamomile, Golden Seal, Lemon Grass, Myrrh, Peppermint, Rose Hips, Sage, Slippery Elm, Yarrow.

5-B   Garlic, Rosehips, Rosemary, Parsley, Watercress.

11-   Capsicum, Ginger, Golden Seal, Licorice.

16-A   Capsicum, Echinacea, Myrrh, Yarrow.

16-B   Capsicum, Echinacea, Golden Seal, Yarrow.

16-C   Plantain, Black Walnut, Golden Seal Root, Bugleweed, Marshmallow, Lobelia.

Vitamins

A, C, E.

Minerals

Calcium.

Diet

Liquids, juices (not orange).

Energizing

Generate; place the coned fingers of one hand on lymphatic node, the other on the following acupressure locations:

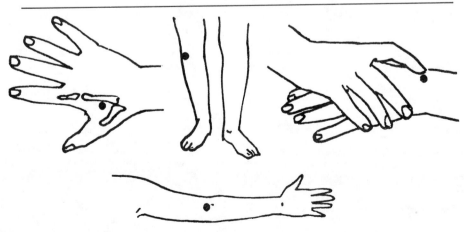

FRACTURES

Herbal Combinations

4-A   Alfalfa, Comfrey, Horsetail, Irish Moss, Lobelia, Oat Straw.

4-B   Horsetail, Comfrey, Oatstraw, Lobelia.

24-A   Aloe Vera, Comfrey, Golden Seal, Slippery Elm.

24-B   Comfrey, White Oak Bark, Mullein, Black Walnut, Marshmallow, Gravel Root, Wormwood, Lobelia, Scullcap.

EMERGENCY: Wrap in combination number three (above) until you can get to a doctor.

Minerals

Calcium, Magnesium.

Diet

Raw or pasteurized milk (not homogenized). Whey (goat whey is best.)

Energizing

Generate; pin point fracture with coned fingers of one hand, place coned fingers of the other hand on lymphatic node. Then continue generating, place coned fingers of one hand on lymphatic node, the other on the following acupressure location:

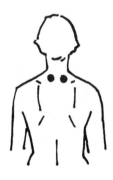

FRIGIDITY
(See also: *Sterility*)

Herbal Combinations

32- Capsicum, Chickweed, Damiana, Echinacea, Garlic, Ginseng, Gotu Kola, Periwinkle, Sarsaparilla, Saw Palmetto.

Damiana, Ginseng, Saw Palmetto - 1 capsule each at every meal.

Vitamins
E, Pantothenic Acid.

Minerals
Zinc.

Diet
Wheat germ, brewer's yeast, lots of dark green, leafy vegetables.

Energizing
Generate; place the coned fingers of one hand on lymphatic node, the other on the following acupressure locations: (#45 of gland chart)

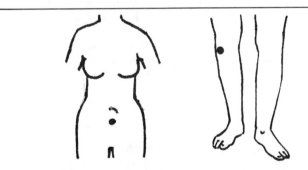

FROST BITE

Herbs

Oat Straw as a wash externally--be gentle.

Energizing

Generate; pin point frostbite with coned fingers of one hand, place the coned fingers of the other hand on lymphatic node.

GALL BLADDER

Herbal Combinations

22-A Angelica, Birch Leaves, Blessed Thistle, Chamomile, Dandelion, Gentian, Golden Rod, Horsetail, Liverwort Leaves, Lobelia, Parsley, Red Beet.

22-B Barberry Bark, Cramp Bark, Fennel, Ginger, Catnip, Peppermint, Wild Yam

Cascara Sagrada.

Vitamins

A, B, C, D, E.

Diet

Three Day Gall Stone Cleanse: Apple juice every day. Each night: ½ cup olive oil and ½ cup lemon juice, before retiring. OR Two days nothing but apple juice, third morning ½ cup olive oil and ½ cup lemon juice plus enema (quite hard on the system).

Enemas

Garlic every morning for three days. (See also: *Enemas*). Take acidophilus night and morning.

Energizing

Think positively, but humbly. Repeat a positive phrase to the rhythm of the bounce. Repeat over and over. Then continue generating, place the coned fingers of one hand on lymphatic node, the other on the following acupressure locations:

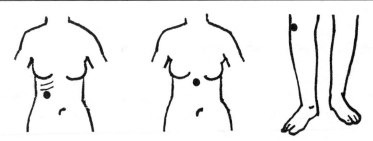

GANGRENE
(See also: *Infection*)

Herbal Combinations

3-A Barberry, Burdock, Cascara Sagrada, Chaparral, Dandelion, Licorice, Red Clover, Sarsaparilla, Yarrow, Yellow Dock.

3-B Red Clover, Chaparral, Licorice, Peach Bark, Oregon Grape, Stilingia, Cascara Sagrada, Sarsaparilla, Prickly Ash Bark, Burdock, Buckthorn.

16-A Capsicum, Echinacea, Myrrh, Yarrow.

16-B Capsicum, Echinacea, Golden Seal, Yarrow.

16-C Plantain, Black Walnut, Golden Seal Root, Bugleweed, Marshmallow, Lobelia.

24-A Aloe Vera, Comfrey, Golden Seal, Slippery Elm.

24-B Comfrey, White Oak Bark, Mullein, Black Walnut, Marshmallow, Gravel Root, Wormwood, Lobelia, Scullcap.

Chamomile--Use as a poultice to prevent gangrene. (See: *Poultice*).

Vitamins

C, E.

Diet

Very little meat. NO red meat.

DANGER! Do Not use the machine for Gangrene.

GAS
(See also: *Colon, Stomach*)

Herbal Combinations

For the Colon:

17- Fennel, Wild Yam, Peppermint, Ginger, Papaya, Spearmint, Catnip, Lobelia.

22-A Angelica, Birch Leaves, Blessed Thistle, Chamomile, Dandelion, Gentian, Golden Rod, Horsetail, Liverwort Leaves, Lobelia, Parsley, Red Beet.

22-B Barberry Bark, Cramp Bark, Fennel, Ginger, Catnip, Peppermint, Wild Yam.

For the Stomach:
Golden Seal and Papaya Mint taken about ½ hour before eating.

Vitamins

B Complex.

Diet

Stay away from fatty, spicy, and acid foods. (See: *Correct Food Combinations*).

Energizing

Generate; place the coned fingers of one hand on lymphatic node, the other on the following acupressure location:

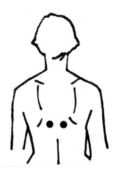

GASTRITIS
(Inflammation of the stomach).
(See also: *Gas and Stomach*).

Herbal Combinations

14- Hops, Scullcap, Valerian Root.

30-A Capsicum, Golden Seal, Myrrh.

30-B Marshmallow, Slippery Elm, Comfrey, Lobelia, Ginger, Wild Yam.

Diet

Neutralize acid by having no coffee, tobacco, alcohol or drugs. If you eat meat, take a protein digestive aid (Betane Hydro-chloric acid and Pepsin).

Energizing

(See: *Stomach*).

GLAUCOMA
(See: *Eyes and Eye Wash*).

GOITER
(See also: *Thyroid*).

Herbal Combinations

19-A Alfalfa, Dandelion, Kelp.

29-A Capsicum, Irish Moss, Kelp, Parsley.

29-B Parsley, Watercress, Kelp, Irish Moss, Sarsaparilla, Black Walnut, Iceland Moss.

Kelp.

Paint throat (goiter area) with natural iodine. (Black Walnut Hulls). This looks terrible, but it gets the needed iodine to the affected area faster (looks better than an ear to ear incision, and you won't have to wear turtlenecks as long!)

Diet

Use a Kelp shaker instead of salt, and put it on everything. You will enjoy the new taste sensations if you can make it through the first week.

Energizing

Generate; pin-pointing Goiter with coned fingers, with other hand place coned fingers on lymphatic node. Then continue generating, place the coned fingers of one hand on lymphatic node and the other on the following acupressure location:

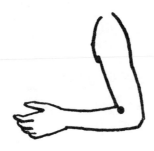

GONORRHEA
(See: *Venereal Disease*).

GRAVEL AND STONES
(See: *Gall Bladder and Kidneys*).

GOUT
(See: *Arthritis and Rheumatism*).

Herbal Combinations

17- Alfalfa, Black Cohosh, Bromalain Powder, Burdock Root, Capsicum, Centaury, Chaparral, Comfrey, Lobelia, Yarrow, Yucca.

4-A Alfalfa, Comfrey, Horsetail, Irish Moss, Lobelia, Oat Straw.

4-B Horstail, Comfrey, Oat Straw, Lobelia.

24-A Aloe Vera, Comfrey, Golden Seal, Slippery Elm.

24-B Comfrey, White Oak Bark, Mullein, Black Walnut, Marshmallow, Gravel Root, Wormwood, Lobelia, Scullcap.

Vitamins

B Complex, C, E.

Minerals

Chelated Calcium, Potassium.

Diet

Eat lots of fish, brown rice and vegetables.

Energizing

(See body parts which are affected).

GUMS

Herbal Combinations

30-A Capsicum, Golden Seal, Myrrh.

30-B Marshmallow, Slippery Elm, Comfrey, Lobelia, Ginger, Wild Yam.

White Oak Bark.

Aloe Vera and/or Myrrh Gum- Rub directly on gums twice a day. Leave it in your mouth to mix with saliva. Hold it in your mouth, working it around your teeth as long as you can stand it.

Vitamins

C, keep increasing doses until your gums quit bleeding. You may have to take huge quantities.

Diet

Raw fruits and vegetables, things to make you chew hard and long. (NOT taffy!)

Energizing

Massage gums while bouncing. Generate; place the coned fingers of one hand on lymphatic node, the other on the following acupressure location:

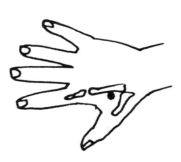

HAIR
(See also: *Baldness, Dandruff*)

Herbal Combinations

4-A Alfalfa, Comfrey, Horsetail, Irish Moss, Lobelia, Oat Straw, - helps split ends.

Yarrow- Retain color.

Jojoba Oil- baldness.

Vitamins

PABA - Retains color.

Energizing

See: *Skin, Dandruff, Baldness.*

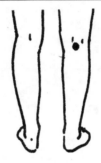

HAND

Energizing

Generate; place the coned fingers of one hand on lymphatic node, the other on the following acupressure locations:

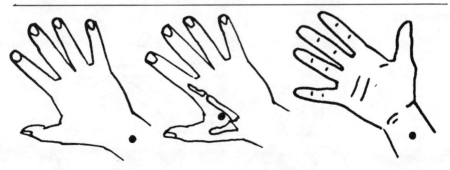

HALITOSIS
(See: *Bad Breath*).

HANGOVER
(See: *Alcoholism*).

HARDENING of the ARTERIES
(See: *Arteriosclerosis*).

HAYFEVER

Herbal Combinations

7 A&B   Bayberry, Eyebright, Golden Seal. (Capsicum optional).

10-A   Black Cohosh, Blessed Thistle, Pleurisy Root, Scullcap.

10-B   Brigham Tea, Marshmallow, Golden Seal Root, Chaparral, Burdock, Parsley, Capsicum, Lobelia.

21-A   Comfrey, Lobelia, Comfrey, Mullein, Slippery Elm.

21-B   Marshmallow, Mullein, Comfrey, Lobelia, Chickweed.

Vitamins

A, C, E.

Minerals

Calcium.

Diet

Eat as many fruits and vegetables as possible. Eat no red meats or dairy products. (See also: *Correct Food Combinations*).

Energizing

Generate; place the coned fingers of one hand on lymphatic node the other on the following acupressure locations:

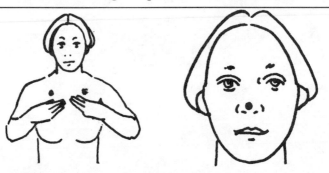

HEADACHE
(See also: *Migraine Headache*).

Herbal Combinations

1-   Capsicum, Valerian Root, Wild Lettuce.

4-A   Alfalfa, Comfrey, Horsetail, Irish Moss, Lobelia, Oat Straw.

4-B   Horsetail, Comfrey, Oat Straw, Lobelia.

Vitamins

B Complex.

Minerals

Calcium.

Enemas

Pure water or Coffee. (See: *Enemas*).

Diet

No coffee, cigarettes, or drugs. (See: *Correct Food Combinations*).

Generate; place the coned fingers of one hand on lymphatic node, the other on the following acupressure locations:

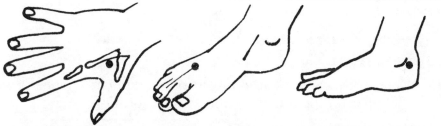

Generate with partner. Place your coned fingers on lymphatic node in chest area. Your partner's coned fingers on the following locations:

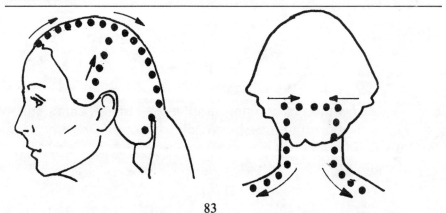

HEARING
(See: *Ears* or *Deafness*).

HEART

Herbal Combinations

4-A Alfalfa, Comfrey, Horsetail, Irish Moss, Lobelia, Oat Straw.

4-B Horsetail, Comfrey, Oatstraw, Lobelia.

13-A Capsicum, Garlic, Hawthorne.

13-B Capsicum, Parsley, Ginger, Garlic, Ginseng, Golden Seal Root.

Hawthorn Extract.

Lobelia - Heart palpitations.

Capsicum - 1 tsp. in 8 oz. pure water. Drink right down, will stop certain heart attacks in from 3 to 20 minutes.

Vitamins

B, E, B Complex, Lecithin.

Minerals

Calcium, Magnesium, Potassium.

Diet

Low fat, low calories, low salt.

Energizing

Generate; place the coned fingers of one hand on lymphatic node, the other on the following acupressure locations:

EMERGENCY POINT
(Palpitation)

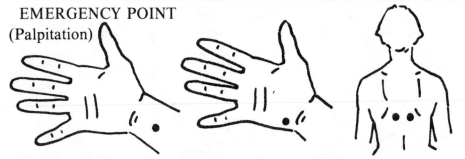

Directed thinking is important when strengthening this area. Control your emotions by saying out loud "God loves me, my husband (wife) loves me, my friends love me," etc., to the rhythm of the bounce. Start with only 30 seconds.

HEARTBURN

Herbal Combinations

4-A Alfalfa, Comfrey, Horsetail, Irish Moss, Lobelia, Oat Straw.

4-B Horsetail, Comfrey, Oat Straw, Lobelia.

17-A Fennel, Wild Yam, Peppermint, Ginger, Papaya, Spearmint, Catnip, Lobelia.

30-A Capsicum, Golden Seal, Myrrh.

30-B Marshmallow, Slippery Elm, Comfrey, Lobelia, Ginger, Wild Yam.

Vitamins

B Complex.

Minerals

Calcium.

Diet

See: *Correct Food Combinations.*

Energizing

Generate; place the coned fingers of one hand on lymphatic node, with the other hand, place coned fingers on pin point of pain. Build up to jumping and jogging.

HEMORRHOIDS or PILES

Herbal Combinations

30-A Capsicum, Golden Seal, Myrrh.

30-B Marshmallow, Slippery Elm, Comfrey, Lobelia, Ginger, Wild Yam.

Golden Seal and White Oak Bark packs reduce swelling.

Vitamins

A, B, C, E, Lecithin.
Vitamin E on a piece or raw potato the size of a suppository; insert at night to reduce swelling and pain.

Minerals

Potassium.

Enemas

Slippery Elm or White Oak Bark. (See: *Enemas*).

Diet

No acids. (Includes Tomato or orange juice).

Energizing

Generate; place the coned fingers of one hand on lymphatic node, the other on the following acupressure locations:

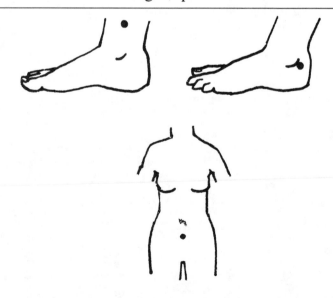

HEPATITIS
(See: *Liver*).

HERPES
(See also: *Mouth Sores*).

Herbs

Myrrh.

White Oak Bark and Golden Seal Tea to rinse and swab mouth and gums.

Aloe Vera - swish in mouth.

Diet

If mouth begins to hurt at all when you start to eat something, DO NOT EAT IT! Usually acids and sugars cause these symptoms.

Energizing

Generate; place the coned fingers of one hand on lymphatic node, and with the coned fingers of the other hand pin point the problem in the mouth or gums.

HICCOUGH

Energizing

Generate; place the coned fingers of one hand on lymphatic node, the other on the following acupressure locations:

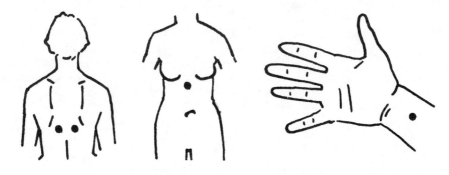

HIGH BLOOD PRESSURE
(See: *Blood Pressure*).

HIVES

Herbs

Aloe Vera - internally and externally.

Generate; place the coned fingers of one hand on lymphatic node, and the other on the following acupressure locations:

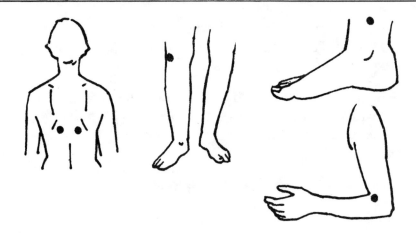

HOARSENESS

Herbal Combinations

21-A   Comfrey, Lobelia, Marshmallow, Mullein, Slippery Elm.

21-B   Marshmallow, Mullein, Comfrey, Lobelia, Chickweed.

Liquid Chlorophyll - use as a gargle.

Vitamins

C, E.

Energizing

Generate; place the coned fingers of one hand on lymphatic node, the coned fingers of the other hand pin pointing the problem, then continue with the following acupressure locations:

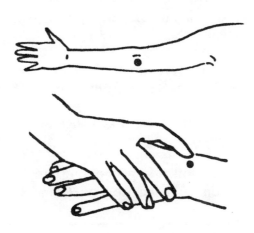

HORMONE IMBALANCE

Herbal Combinations

Female Imbalance

Dong Quai.

8-A   Blessed Thistle, Capsicum, Ginger, Golden Seal, Gravel Root, Lobelia, Marshmallow, Parsley, Raspberry.

8-B   Black Cohosh, Sarsaparilla, Ginseng, Licorice, False Unicorn, Blessed Thistle, Squawvine.

32-   Capsicum, Chickweed, Damiana, Echinacea, Garlic, Ginseng, Gotu Kola, Periwinkle, Sarsaparilla, Saw Palmetto.

Male Imbalance

26-A   Black Cohosh, Capsicum, Ginger, Golden Seal, Gotu Kola, Kelp, Licorice, Lobelia.

32-   Capsicum, Chickweed, Damiana, Echinacea, Garlic, Ginseng, Gotu Kola, Periwinkle, Sarsaparilla, Saw Palmetto.

Ginseng and Sarsaparilla are taken together.

Energizing

Generate; place the coned fingers of one hand on lymphatic node, the other hand on # 45 location on Gland Chart. (See: *Gland Chart*).

HYPERACTIVITY

Herbal Combinations

4-A   Alfalfa, Comfrey, Horsetail, Irish Moss, Lobelia, Oat Straw.

4-B   Horsetail, Comfrey, Oat Straw, Lobelia.

6-B   Black Cohosh, Calsicum, Ginger, Hops, Mistletoe, Lobelia, Scullcap, Wood Betony, Lady's Slipper, Valerian.

Licorice.

Lobelia.

Vitamins

B Complex.

Minerals

Massive doses of all minerals.

Diet

Avoid ALL Artificial flavoring and food coloring. (See: *Food Best for Human Consumption*).

Energizing

Let patient use machine any time with arms away from body.

HYPOGLYCEMIA

Herbal Combinations

4-A Alfalfa, Comfrey, Horsetail, Irish Moss, Lobelia, Oat Straw.

4-B Horsetail, Comfrey, Oat Straw, Lobelia.

15- Dandelion, Licorice, Horseradish, Safflowers.

23-A Bistort, Blueberry Leaves, Buchu, Capsicum, Comfrey, Dandelion, Garlic, Golden Seal, Juniper Berries, Licorice, Marshmallow, Mullein, Uva-Ursi, Yarrow.

23-B Juniper Berries, Uva Ursi, Licorice, Mullein, Capsicum, Golden Seal Root.

25- Capsicum, Red Clover, Soy.

BE CAREFUL OF GOLDEN SEAL.

Safflowers are good to take before energizing.

Vitamins

B Complex, C, E, Pantothenic Acid.

Minerals

Magnesium, Potassium.

Diet

See: *Hypoglycemia Diet.*

Energizing

Directed thinking is important when strengthening this area. Control your emotions by saying aloud: "God loves me, my husband (wife) loves me, my friends love me," etc., to the rhythm of the bounce. Start with only 30 seconds.

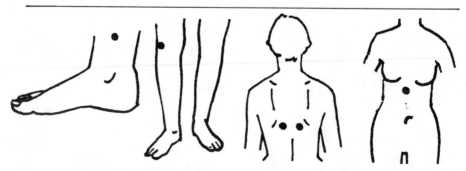

HYPOTHALMUS

Energizing

Generate; think of very pleasant thoughts. If you can't think of any, repeat the 23rd Psalm to the ryhthm of the bounce. Place the coned fingers of one hand on lymphatic node. Place the coned fingers of the other hand on location # 1 on the Gland Chart. (See: *Gland Chart* page 203.)

HYSTERIA

Herbal Combinations

4-A   Alfalfa, Comfrey, Horsetail, Irish Moss, Lobelia, Oat Straw.

6-A   Black Cohosh, Capsicum, Ginger, Hops, Mistletoe, St. Johnswort, Valerian, Wood Betony.

14-   Hops, Scullcap, Valerian Root.

Lobelia Extract for quick results.

Vitamins

B Complex.

Minerals

Calcium

Diet

Little or no sugar or refined starches. (See: *Correct Food Combinations* page 189).

Energizing

Generate; place the coned fingers of one hand on lymphatic node, place coned fingers of the other hand on the following acupressure locations:

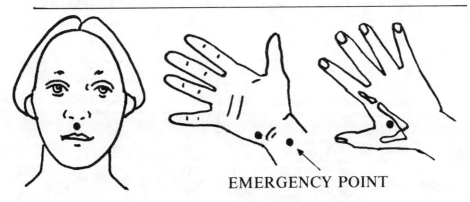

EMERGENCY POINT

93

IMPOTENCY
(See: *Frigidity*).

INDIGESTION
(See: *Digestion*)

INFECTION

Herbal Combinations

3-A   Barberry, Burdock, Cascara Sagrada, Chaparral, Dandelion, Licorice, Red Clover, Sarsaparilla, Yarrow, Wellow Dock.

3-B   Red Clover, Chaparral, Licorice, Peach Bark, Oregon Grape, Stillingia, Cascara Sagrada, Sarsaparilla, Prickly Ash Bark, Burdock, Buckthorn.

16-A   Capsicum, Echinacea, Myrrh, Yarrow.

16-B   Capsicum, Echinacea, Golden Seal, Yarrow.

16-C   Plantain, Black Walnut, Golden Seal Root, Bugleweed, Marshmallow, Lobelia.

24-A   Aloe Vera, Comfrey, Golden Seal, Slippery Elm. (Used also externally).

24-B   Comfrey, White Oak Bark, Mullein, Black Walnut, Marshmallow, Gravel Root, Wormwood, Lobelia, Scullcap.

Vitamins

A, C, E.

Douches

Capsicum and Garlic. (See: *Douche*).

Energizing

Generate; place the coned fingers of one hand on lymphatic node, place the coned fingers of the other hand on the following acupressure locations:

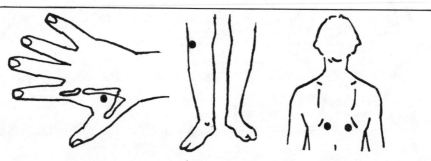

INFLAMMATION and SWELLING
(See also: *Bruises*)

Herbal Combinations

3-A   Barberry, Burdock, Cascara Sagrada, Chaparral, Dandelion, Licorice, Red Clover, Sarsaparilla, Yarrow, Yellow Dock.

24-A   Aloe Vera, Comfrey, Golden Seal, Slippery Elm. (Use also externally).

24-B   Comfrey, White Oak Bark, Mullein, Black Walnut, Marshmallow, Gravel Root, Wormwood, Lobelia, Scullcap. (Use externally).

Comfrey and Wood Betony or Onion packs are good for sprains.

Vitamins

A, C, E.

Energizing

Generate; place the coned fingers of one hand on lymphatic node, the coned fingers of the other hand to pin point the inflammed area.

INSANITY

Herbal Combinations

6-A   Black Cohosh, Capsicum, Ginger, Hops, Mistletoe, St. Johnswort, Valerian, Wood Betony.

6-B   Black Cohosh, Capsicum, Hops, Mistletoe, Lobelia, Scullcap, Wood Betony, Lady's Slipper, Valerian.

12-A   Capsicum, Ginseng, Gotu Kola.

14-   Hops, Scullcap, Valerian Root.

Vitamins

B Complex, Pantothenic Acid, large amounts.

Diet

(See: *Correct Food Combinations* page 189).

Energizing

Generate; place the coned fingers of both hands on lymphatic nodes in chest area, then at temple area. Repeat aloud: "I feel healthy, I feel happy, I feel terrific!" in rhythm with the bounce. If impossible to say, have partner repeat it.

INSECT BITES
(See: *Bee Stings and Bites*).

INSOMNIA

Herbal Combinations

4-A   Alfalfa, Comfrey, Horsetail, Irish Moss, Lobelia, Oat Straw.

4-B   Horsetail, Comfrey, Oat Straw, Lobelia.

6-A   Black Cohosh, Capsicum, Ginger, Hops, Mistletoe, St. Johnswort, Valerian, Wood Betony.

6-B   Black Cohosh, Capsicum, Hops, Mistletoe, Lobelia, Scullcap, Wood Betony, Lady's Slipper, Valerian.

14-   Hops, Scullcap, Valerian Root.

Vitamins

B Complex - large amounts, add Fennel to cut appetite.

Minerals

Calcium, Iron, Zinc.

Diet

See: *Correct Food Combinations*

Energizing

Generate; place the coned fingers of one hand on lymphatic node, the coned fingers of the other hand on the following acupressure locations:

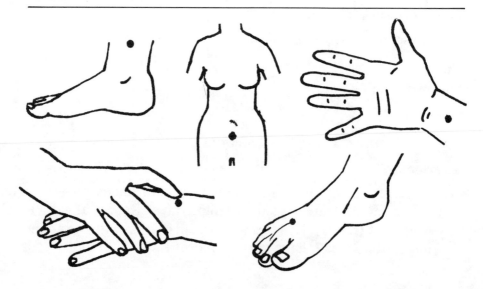

INTESTINES
(See also: *Colon, Constipation, Diarrhea, Bowel*).

Inflammation
Energizing
Generate; place the coned fingers of one hand on lymphatic node, place coned fingers of the other hand on the following acupressure locations:

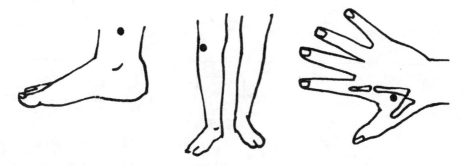

Small Intestines:
Energizing
Generate; place the coned fingers of one hand on lymphatic node, place coned fingers of the other hand *stroking* the following area. Positive thinking is important here. Repeat "God appreciates me, my husband (wife) appreciates me, my children appreciate me, I appreciate myself..." or some other positive phrase, scripture, or saying of your choice, to the rhythm of the bounce.

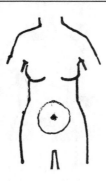

Large Intestine

Energizing

Generate; place the coned fingers of one hand on lymphatic node, use the coned fingers of the other hand to *stroke* the following area. Repeat, "I live in moderation, I am good natured, I am meek, and the meek will inherit the earth!" to the rhythm of the bounce.

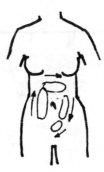

Ascending Colon

Energizing

Generate; place the coned fingers of one hand on lymphatic node, and use the coned fingers of the other hand to *stroke* the following area. Repeat: "I am not lonely, God is with me, my family is with me, my friends are only as far away as the telephone..." to the rhythm of the bounce.

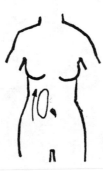

(Continued)

Transverse Colon

Energizing

Continue generating, *stroking* the following area. Repeat: "I am certain of my well-being, I believe that God loves me, I believe my family loves me, I believe my friends love me..."

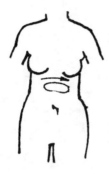

Descending Colon

Energizing

Continue generating, *stroking the following area. Repeat: "God includes me in his plan, my family includes me in their plans, my friends include me in their plans," etc., to the rhythm of the bounce.*

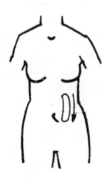

(Intestines continued)

Sigmoid Colon

Energizing

Generate; place the coned fingers of one hand on lymphatic node, use the coned fingers of the other hand to *stroke* the following area. Repeat, "I am not at my wit's end, I will find an answer, there is always a solution!" in rhythm with the bounce.

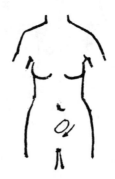

ITCHING

(See also: *Eczema, Shin Disease, Vagina*).

Herbal Combinations

3-A   Barberry, Burdock, Cascara Sagrada, Chaparral, Dandelion, Licorice, Red Clover, Sarsaparilla, Yarrow, Yellow Dock.

3-B   Red Clover, Chaparral, Licorice, Poke Root, Peach Bark, Oregon Grape, Stillingia, Cascara Sagrada, Sarsaparilla, Prickly Ash Bark, Burdock, Buckthorn.

Chickweed.

Yellow Dock.

Aloe Vera.

Vitamins

B Complex.

Minerals

Calcium, Zinc.

Energizing

Generate; place the coned fingers of one hand on lymphatic node, the coned fingers of the other hand on the following acupressure location:

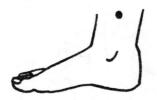

JAUNDICE

Herbal Combinations

3-A Barberry, Burdock, Cascara Sagrada, Chaparral, Dandelion, Licorice, Red Clover, Sarsaparilla, Yarrow, Yellow Dock.

3-B Red Clover, Chaparral, Licorice, Peach Bark, Oregon Grape, Stillingia, Cascara Sagrada, Sarsaparilla, Prickly Ash Bark, Burdock, Buckthorn.

22-A Angelica, Birch Leaves, Blessed Thistle, Chamonile, Dandelion, Gentian, Golden Rod, Horsetail, Liverwort Leaves, Lobelia, Parsley, Red Beet.

22-B Barberry Bark, Cramp Bark, Fennel, Ginger, Catnip, Peppermint, Wild Yam.

Cascara Sagrada.

Vitamins

B, C, E.

Energizing

Generate; place the coned fingers of one hand on lymphatic node,m place coned fingers of the other hand on the following acupressure locations:

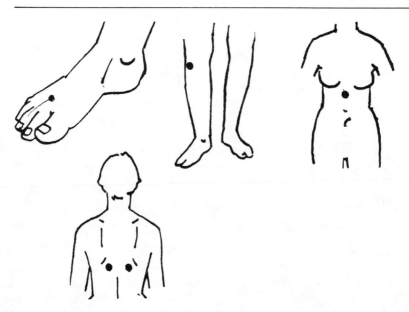

102

JOINTS

(See: *Arthritis, Gout, Rheumatism,* and specific joints.)

KNEE

Energizing

Generate; place the coned fingers of one hand on lymphatic node, use the coned fingers of the other hand to *stroke* and pin point the pain.

KIDNEYS

(See also: *Bladder, Urination*).

Herbal Combinations

18-A Chamomile, Dandelion, Juniper, Parsley, Uva-Ursi.

18-B Juniper Berries, Parsley, Uva-Ursi, Marshmallow, Lobelia, Ginger, Golden Seal Root, .

19-A Alfalfa, Dandelion, Kelp.

23-B Capsicum, Uva-Ursi, Parsley, Golden Seal Root, Gravel Root, Juniper Berries, Marshmallow, Ginger, Ginseng.

Catnip, Oat Straw amd Parsley may help dissolve kidney stones.

Vitamins

A, B, C, E.

Minerals

Magnesium, Zinc.

Diet

Lemon juice takes the edge off kidney stones.

Enema

Capsicum. (See also: *Enemas*).

Energizing

Generate; plave the coned fingers of one hand on lymphatic node, place the coned fingers of the other hand on the following acupressure locations. Repeat, "I am reliable, I am devoted and I am faithful to the imporatnt things in life!" in rhythm with the bounce.

(Illustrations next page...)

(illustrations, Kidney.)

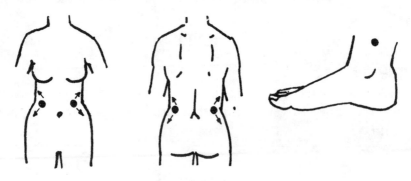

LABOR
(See also: *Afterpain, Pregnancy*).

Energizing

DANGER! Do not do this *during* pregnancy, ONLY when ready to deliver.

Generate; place the coned fingers of on hand on lymphatic node, the other on the following acupressure location:

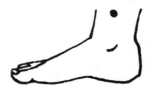

LACTATION

Herbal Combinations

Enrich:
4-A Alfalfa, Comfrey, Horsetail, Irish Moss, Lobelia, Oat Straw.

Blessed Thistle.

To promote:
Marshmallow, Raspberry, Beer.

Slow Down:
Parsley, Sage.
Add Papaya to cow's milk to resemble breast milk.

Minerals

Calcium, Manganese, Phosphorus.

Diet

See: *Food Best for Human Consumption.* Page 190.

Energizing

See: *Breast.*

LARYNGITIS
(See: Hoarseness).

LEARNING DISABILITIES

Herbal Combinations

6-A   Black Cohosh, Capsicum, Ginger, Hops, Mistletoe, St. Johnswort, Valerian, Wood Betony.

6-B   Black Cohosh, Capsicum, Hops, Mistletoe, Lobelia, Scullcap, Wood Betony, Lady's Slipper, Valerian.

4-A   Alfalfa, Comfrey, Horsetail, Irish Moss, Lobelia, Oat Straw (large amounts).

Vitamins

Natural multiple vitamin.

Minerals

Natural multiple mineral.

Diet

Keep all sugar from the diet. Keep a diary of when the child's mind seems to be the slowest, see what he has eaten previous to this time, and keep those foods out of the diet.

Energizing

As a child is jumping with both feet in the air at a time, have him keep repeating what has to be learned in rhythm with his jumps. The strongest learning force is when he is at the bottom of the jump. Example: B says bŭ, bŭ, bŭ,...

C says kŭ, kŭ, kŭ,...etc.

LEG

Energizing

Generate; place the coned fingers of one hand on lymphatic node, with the coned fingers of the other hand, pin point pain, then on the following acupressure locations:

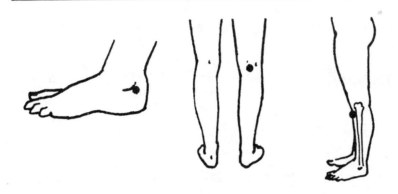

LEUCORRHEA
A discharge from the vagina.

Herbal Combinations

35- Squawvine, Chickweed, Slippery Elm, Comfrey, Yellow Dock, Golden Seal Root, Mullein, Marshmallow.

Vitamins

A, B, C, E, Pantothenic Acid.

Minerals

Calcium, Zinc.

Diet

Absolutely no sweets, alcohol, coffee or tea.

Douches

See above herbal combination. (See also: *Douche*).

Energizing

Generate; place the coned fingers of one hand on lymphatic node, placed coned fingers of the other hand on location # 45 of Gland Chart. (Page 203). If no result comes from generating, then jump with both feet off machine, coned fingers remaining on the same spot.

LICE

Herbal Combinations

3-A Alfalfa, Comfrey, Horsetail, Irish Moss, Lobelia, Oat Straw.

3-B Black Cohosh, Blessed Thistle, Pleurisy Root, Scullcap.

Liquid Chlorophyll.

Juniper Berries for itching - internal and external.

Vitamins

B Complex all year around if head lice are known to be in the area.

Minerals

Calcium, Magnesium.

Diet

As many dark green vegetables as you can get down. Smaller amounts of meats and sweets.

Energizing

(See: *Nerves* and *Itching*).

LIVER
(See also: *Jaundice*).

Herbal Combinations

3-A Barberry, Burdock, Cascara Sagrada. Chaparral, Dandelion, Licorice, Red Clover, Sarsaparilla, Yarrow, Yellow Dock.

22-A Angelica, Birch Leaves, Blessed Thistle, Chamomile, Dandelion, Gentian, Golden Rod, Horsetail, Liverwort Leaves, Lobelia, Parsley, Red Beet.

22-B Barberry Bark, Cramp Bark, Fennel, Ginger, Catnip, Peppermint, Wild Yam.

Vitamins

A, B, C, E.

Minerals

Coffee, Capsicum. (See: *Enemas*).

Energizing

Generate; place the coned fingers of one hand on lymphatic node, place the coned fingers of the other hand on the following acupressure locations. Repeat: "I feel healthy, I feel happy, I feel satisfied!" to the rhythm of the bounce.

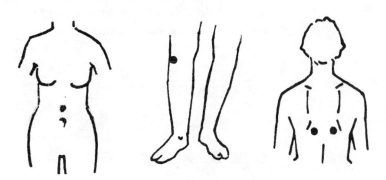

LOCK JAW
(See: *Tetanus*).

LONGEVITY
(See also: *Vitality*)

Herbal Combinations

12-A Capsicum, Ginseng, Gotu Kola.

32- Capsicum, Chickweed, Damiana, Echinacea, Garlic, Ginseng, Gotu Kola, Periwinkle, Sarsaparilla, Saw Palmetto.

Bee Pollen.

Aloe Vera.

Ginseng.

Vitamins

A, B, C, E.

A natutal multiple vitamin.

Diet

(See: *Foods Best for Human Consumption*).

Energizing

Use all three forms of exercise; Health, strength, and jogging for a feeling of well being and vibrant countenance.

LOW BLOOD PRESSURE
(See: *Blood Pressure*).

LOW BLOOD SUGAR
(See: *Hypoglycemia*).

LUMBAGO
(See: *Back; lower, Cramps; leg and muscle, Rheumatism.*)

LUNGS
(See: *Emphysema, Pneumonia*).

LUPUS
(See also: *Arthritis, Skin Disease*)

Herbal Combinations

2-B Alfalfa, Black Cohosh, Bromalain Powder, Burdock Root, Capsicum, Centaury, Chaparral, Comfrey, Lobelia, Yarrow, Yucca.

3-A Barberry, Burdock, Cascara Sagrada, Chaparral, Dandelion, Licorice, Red Clover, Sarsaparilla, Yarrow, Yellow Dock.

4-A Alfalfa, Comfrey, Horsetail, Irish Moss, Lobelia, Oat Straw.

6-A Black Cohosh, Capsicum, Ginger, Hops, Mistletoe, St. Johnswort, Valerian, Wood Betony.

18-A Chamomile, Dandelion, Juniper, Parsley, Uva-Ursi.

Black Walnut.

Vitamins

A, E, and high doses of B, and C.

Diet

A cleansing diet *The Herbalist Magazine* April 1978 pp. 24-25. Eliminate sugars and red meat out completely. Eat lots of fruit, vegetables, nuts and juices.

Enemas

Garlic once a week. (See also: *Enemas*). Note: You will feel worse for a month or so until toxins leave the body, but stick with it!

Energizing

See: *Arthritis*

LYMPH AND SWOLLEN GLANDS

Herbal Combinations

3-A Barberry, Burdock, Cascara Sagrada, Chaparral, Dandelion, Licorice, Red Clover, Sarsaparilla, Yarrow, Yellow Dock.

16-A Capsicum, Echinacea, Myrrh, Yarrow.

16-B Capsicum, Echinacea, Golden Seal, Yarrow.

Saw Palmetto.

Vitamins

A, C, E, Pantothenic Acid.

Diet

No preservatives, artificial colors or flavors, and chemical foods. (See also: *Food Best for Human Consumption*).

Energizing

Must start out very easy because you may feel dizziness. Get off machine when dizziness occurs, but keep coming back to it. Generate; place the coned fingers of both hands on the lymphatic nodes of the chest area. Breathe in through your nose and out through your mouth. Concentrate on cleaning the toxins out. Repeat: "Out sick toxins, in good health!" to the rhythm of the bounce.

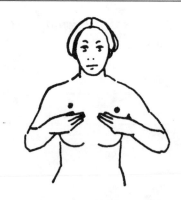

MASTITIS
(See also: *Breast*).

Herbs

Plantain.

Marshmallow.

Chamomile.

Hops.

Diet

Dark, leafy green vegetables, steamed.

Energizing

Generate; place the coned fingers of one hand on lymphatic node, use the coned fingers of the other hand to pin point the distressed area, then on the following acupressure locations:

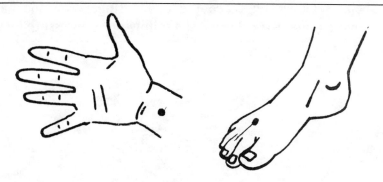

MEASLES

Herbs

Lobelia.

Capsicum.

Red Raspberry.

Tea - 1tsp. Pleurisy Root, ½ tsp. Ginger steeped in 1 pint boiling pure water.

Diet

Plenty of liquids, pure water, vegetable juice, fruit juice and potassium broth. (See also: *Potassium Broth*).

Enemas

Catnip. (See also: *Enemas*).

Energizing

Rubella - Generate; place the coned fingers of one hand on lymphatic node, the other on the following acupressure locations:

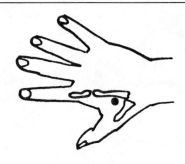

MENIERE'S SYNDROME

(See also: *Ear, Deafness*).

Herbal Combinations

27- Chickweed, Black Cohosh, Golden Seal, Lobelia, Scullcap, Brigham Tea, Licorice.

Use internally or as an ear wash. (See: *Deafness*).

Diet

See: *Food Best for Human Consumption.*

Energizing

Generate; place the coned fingers of one hand on lymphatic node, place the coned fingers of the other hand pin pointing the ear, then on the following acupressure locations:

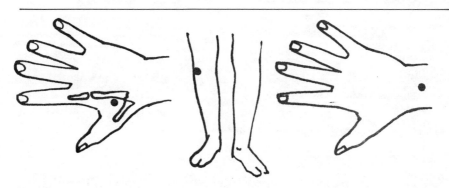

MENOPAUSE

Herbal Combinations

6-A   Black Cohosh, Capsicum, Ginger, Hops, Mistletoe, St. Johnswort, Valerian, Wood Betony.

Blessed Thistle, Capsicum, Ginger, Golden Seal, Gravel Root, Lobelia, Marshmallow, Parsley, Raspberry.

8-B   Black Cohosh, Sarsaparilla, Ginseng, Licorice, False Unicorn, Blessed Thistle, Squawvine.

32-   Capsicum, Chickweed, Damiana, Echinacea, Garlic, Ginseng, Gotu Kola, Periwinkle, Sarsaparilla, Saw Palmetto.

Dong Quai.

Vitamins

A, B, C, E.

Minerals

Calcium, Magnesium, Zinc.

Energizing

Generate; place the coned fingers of one hand on lymphatic node, place the coned fingers of the other hand pin pointing location # 45 on Gland Chart (See: Gland Chart pp. 203), then on the following acupressure locations: (See: *Menstration Difficulties*).

MENSTRUATION
(See also: *Cramps*)

Difficulties

Herbal Combinations

1- Capsicum, Valerian Root, Wild Lettuce.

4-A Alfalfa, Comfrey, Horsetail, Irish Moss, Lobelia, Oat Straw.

4-B Horsetail, Comfrey, Oat Straw, Lobelia.

8-A Blessed Thistle, Capsicum, Ginger, Golden Seal, Gravel Root, Lobelia, Marshmallow, Parsley, Raspberry.

8-B Black Cohosh, Sarsaparilla, Ginseng, Licorice, False Unicorn, Blessed Thistle, Squawvine.

Vitamins

B, C, E.

Minerals

Iron.

Energizing

Generate; place the coned fingers of one hand on lymphatic node, place the coned fingers of the other hand on the following acupressure locations:

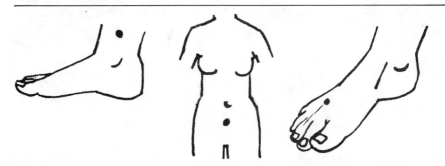

(Continued)

(Continued from previous page).

Excessive

Herbal Combinations

8-A Blessed Thistle, Capsicum, Ginger, Golden Seal, Gravel Root, Lobelia, Marshmallow, Parsley, Raspberry.

8-B Golden Seal Root, Blessed Thistle, Capsicum, Uva-Ursi, Cramp Bark, False Unicorn, Red Raspberry, Sqauwvine, Ginger.

Mistletoe.

Vitamins

B, C, E.

Minerals

Calcium, Iron.

Energizing

Generate; place the coned fingers of one hand on lymphatic node, place the coned fingers of the other hand on the following acupressure locations:

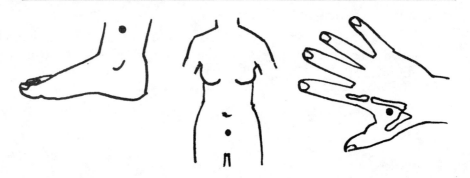

(Continued)

(Continued from previous page).

Supressed

Herbal Combinations

8-A   Blessed Thistle, Capsicum, Ginger, Golden Seal, Gravel Root, Lobelia, Marshmallow, Parsley, Raspberry.

8-B   Black Cohosh, Sarsaparilla, Ginseng, Licorice, False Unicorn, Blessed Thistle, Squawvine.

Dong Quai.

Chamomile.

Vitamins

B, C, E.

Minerals

Iron.

Energizing

Generate; place the coned fingers of one hand on lymphatic node, place the coned fingers of the other hand on the following acupressure locations.

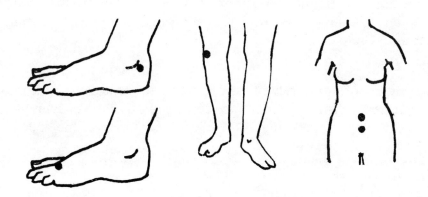

MIGRAINE HEADACHES
(See also: *Headaches*).

Herbal Combinations

4-A   Alfalfa, Comfrey, Horsetail, Irish Moss, Lobelia, Oat Straw.

6-A   Black Cohosh, Capsicum, Ginger, Hops, Mistletoe, St. Johnswort, Valerian, Wood Betony.

6-B   Black Cohosh, Capsicum, Hops, Mistletoe, Lobelia, Scullcap, Wood Betony, Lady's Slipper, Valerian.

Fenugreek.

Lobelia.

Vitamins

B Complex.

Minerals

Calcium.

Diet

No coffee, sugar, or acids.

Enemas

Cleansing, Coffee (See: *Enemas*). IMPORTANT: when you feel the headache coming on, the enema is the first thing you do if you are at home. If you are out, run cold water on your wrists, then hot water. Continue this until you feel normal, but take the enema as soon as possible.

Energizing

Very important to relax first while you are generating, soft music may help. Then place the coned fingers of one hand on lyumphatic node, place coned fingers of the other hand on the following acupressure locations:

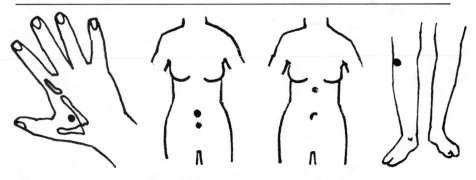

MILK
(See: *Lactation*).

MISCARRIAGE

Herbs

Catnip.

False Unicorn.

Lobelia.

Vitamins

E.

Diet

Lots of green, leafy vegetables, and wheat germ. Keep the calories down. (See also: *Correct Food Combinations, pp.* 189).

Energizing

CAUTION -- be careful where you place your hands, you can start labor! (See: *Labor*). Begin with small walking or shuffling steps. Check heart beat. 140 beats per minute is a good rate. Kick legs to front, side, and back to build up abdominal muscles. You can lie on your back and generate if you don't feel like standing.

MORNING SICKNESS
(See also: *Nausea*)

Herbal Combinations

8-A Blessed Thistle, Capsicum, Ginger, Golden Seal, Gravel Root, Lobelia, Marshmallow, Parsley, Raspberry.

8-B Black Cohosh, Sarsaparilla, Ginseng, Licorice, False Unicorn, Blessed Thistle, Squawvine.

Alfalfa.

Raspberry.

Vitamins

B, E.

Minerals

Calcium.

Diet

High fiber: raw bran, wheat germ, raw vegetables.

Energizing

Start out very slowly, use soft music to help you relax. If you get dizzy, get off and walk around for awhile, then keep coming back to the machine. Place the coned fingers of both hands on the lymphatic nodes in the chest area. NOT on the GROIN.

MOTION SICKNESS

Herbal Combinations

4-A Alfalfa, Comfrey, Horsetail, Irish Moss, Lobelia, Oat Straw.

37- Extract of Chickweed, Black Cohosh, Golden Seal, Lobelia, Scullcap, Brigham Tea, Licorice (See: *Deafness*). Note: Motion Sickness is many times caused by inner ear problems.

Vitamins

A natural multi-vitamin.

Minerals

Calcium.

Diet

Keep something to munch on to keep the ear opened; whole wheat crackers would be good.

Energizing

Before your trip, generate; place coned fingers of one hand on lymphatic node, place the coned fingers of the other hand on the following acupressure locations:

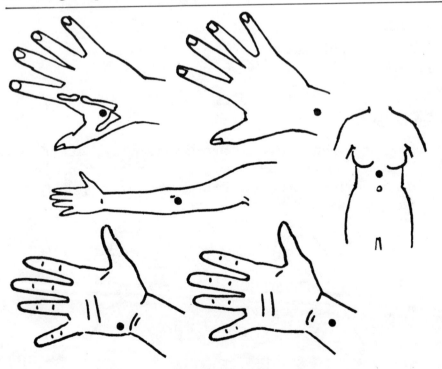

MOUTH SORES
(See: *Gums*).

MUCOUS MEMBRANES AND MUCOUS
(See also: *Sinus*).

Herbal Combinations

4-A Alfalfa, Comfrey, Horstail, Irish Moss, Lobelia, Oat Straw.

6-A Alfalfa, Dandelion, Kelp.

28-A Barberry, Black Walnut, Catnip, Chickweed, Comfrey, Cyani Flowers, Dandelion, Echinacea, Fenugreek, Gentian, Golden Seal, Irish Moss, Mandrake, Myrrh Gum, Pink Root, Safflowers, St. Johnswort, Yellow Dock.

Note: One day take the previous combination, the next day take the following combination: (Continue sequence for 2 weeks.)

28-B Cascara Sagrada, Comfrey, Culver's Root, Mandrake, Mullein, Pumpkin Seeds, Slippery Elm, Violet Leaves, Witch Hazel.

Liquid Chlorophyll.

Vitamins

B, C, E. Natural multi-vitamin, Lecithin.

Minerals

Natural multi-mineral.

Diet

Low on dairy products.

Energizing

Very important to use the machine many times during the day. Place coned fingers on lymphatic nodes in chest, then place rest of hand, fingers extended over the lung area. Generate; then jump; then jog with your hands in place.

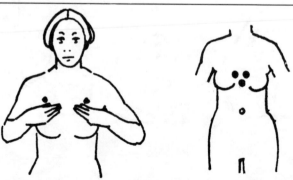

MULTIPLE SCLEROSIS

Herbal Combinations

4-A   Alfalfa, Comfrey, Horsetail, Irish Moss, Lobelia, Oat Straw.

19-A   Alfalfa, Dandelion, Kelp.

28-A   Barberry, Black Walnut, Catnip, Chickweed, Comfrey, Cyani Flowers, Dandelion, Echinacea, Fenugreek, Gentian, Golden Seal Irish Moss, Mandrake, Myrrh Gum, Pink Root, Safflowers, St. Johnswort, Yellow Dock.

   Note: Take the previous combination one day, and take the following combination the next day. Do not take both in the same day.

28-B   Cascara Sagrada, Comfrey, Culver's Root, Mandrake, Mullein, Pumpkin Seeds, Slippery Elm, Violet Leaves, Witch Hazel.

Vitamins

B, C, E. Natural multi-vitamin, Lecithin (huge amounts).

Minerals

Natural multi-mineral, very important.

Diet

Extremely important (See: *Correct Food Combinations*). All vegetables raw or steamed. DO NOT SMOKE OR DRINK ALCOHOL. With this disease you will lose up to 65% of the nutrients you take in, they just go up in smoke!

Energizing

Use soft music to relax. Hold onto the wall to get your balance, or if unable to stand, sit with your feet on the machine and have your partner generate for you. Concentrate on your hands, or a part of your body which is affected. When you have your balance, close your eyes awhile. When you feel dizzy, get off for awhile, but keep coming back to the machine until you can build up your time and gradually begin to exercise with it.

MUSCLES

Herbal Combinations

38- Siberian Ginseng Rootbark, Ho Shou Wu, Black Walnut Hulls, Licorice Root, Gentian Root, Comfrey Root, Fennel Seeds, Bee Pollen, Bayberry Rootbark, Myrrh Gum, Peppermint Leaves, Safflower Flowers, Eucalyptus Leaves, Lemongrass Herb and Capsicum Fruit.

Diet

See: *Foods Best for Human Consumption.*

Energizing

Use jumping for strength, both feet off the machine at once. Then jogging, build up your time (2 minutes is like jogging five miles). You can use dumb bells or weights around wrists and ankles to build the muscles quicker, but build up slowly unless you enjoy being sore. Always finish with fingers on lymphatic nodes to get rid of lactic acids which make sore muscles.

MUSTARD PLASTER

Mild
May be left on overnight - also used for babies. 1 Tblsp. Ginger, 1 Tblsp. Dry Mustard, 1 Tblsp. turpentine, 1 Tblsp. Salt, 3 Tblsp. Lard or Shortening.

Regular
1 Tblsp. Mustard, 3 Tblsp. Flour.
Mix with water, leave on until skin is pink. Note: 1 egg may be added to prevent blisters.

NAUSEA
(See also: *Morning Sickness, Vomiting*).

Herbal Combinations

4-A   Alfalfa, Comfrey, Horsetail, Irish Moss, Lobelia, Oat Straw.

4-B   Horsetail, Oat Straw, Comfrey, Lobelia.

11-   Capsicum, Ginger, Golden Seal, Licorice,
       Raspberry.

Vitamins

B Complex.

Minerals

Calcium.

Energizing

Generate; place the coned fingers of one hand on lymphatic node, the other on the following acupressure locations.

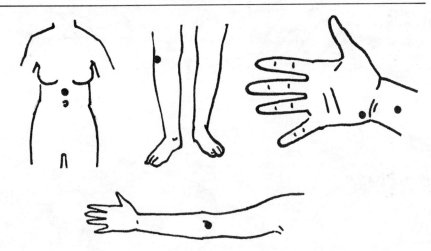

NECK

Herbs

Alfalfa

Minerals

Calcium.

Energizing

Generate; place the coned fingers of one hand on lymphatic node, the other on the following acupressure locations:

STIFF NECK:

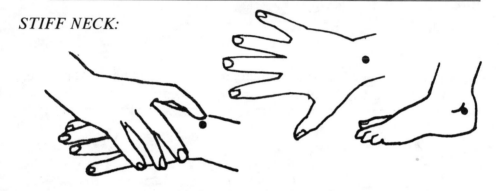

WHIPLASH:

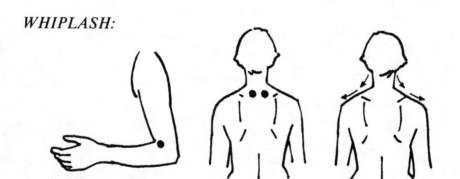

NEPHRITIS
(See: *Kidneys*).

NERVES AND NERVOUS SYSTEM

Herbal Combinations

4-A Alfalfa, Comfrey, Horstail, Irish Moss, Lobelia, Oat Straw.

6-A Black Cohosh, Capsicum, Ginger, Hops, Mistletoe, St. Johnswort, Valerian, Wood Betony.

6-B Black Cohosh, Capsicum, Hops, Mistletoe, Lobelia, Scullcap, Wood Betony, Lady's Slipper, Valerian.

Hops, Scullcap, Valerian Root.

Vitamins

Large doses of B Complex. (Take Fennel to curb your appetite).

Minerals

Calcium, Iodine, Magnesium.

Diet

Cut down on sugar, acids, coffee, tea (drink herbal teas), and smoking. (See also: *Food Best for Human Consumption,* pp. 190).

Energizing

Generate; place the coned fingers of one hand on lymphatic node, the other on the following acupressure locations:

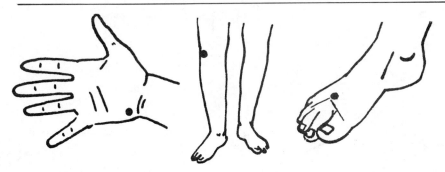

NEURALGIA
(See also: *Nerves*).

Painful condition in the nerve due to some inknown irritation or inflammation.

Energizing

Generate; place the coned fingers of one hand on lymphatic node, the other on the following acupressure locations:

LOWER BACK:

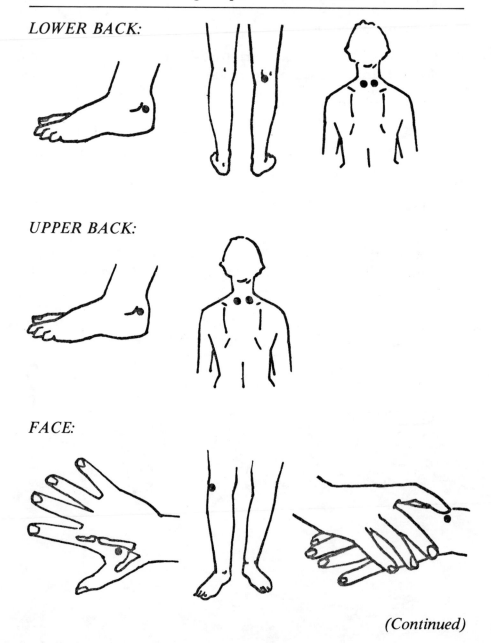

UPPER BACK:

FACE:

(Continued)

JOINT:

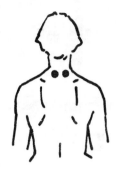

LOWER LIMBS:

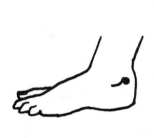 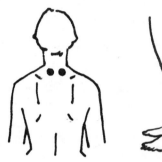 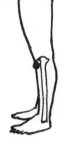

UPPER LIMBS:

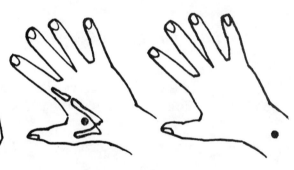

NECK AND BACK OF HEAD:

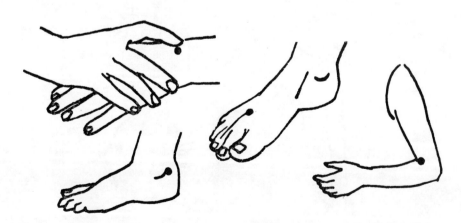

NIGHTMARES

Herbal Combinations

4-A Alfalfa, Comfrey, Horsetail, Irish Moss, Lobelia, Oat Straw.

6-A Black Cohosh, Capsicum, Ginger, Hops, Mistletoe, St. Johnswort, Valerian, Wood Betony.

6-B Black Cohosh, Capsicum, Hops, Mistletoe, Lobelia, Scullcap, Wood Betony, Lady's Slipper, Valerian.

14- Hops, Scullcap, Valerian Root.

Hops.

Vitamins

B Complex.

Minerals

Calcium.

Diet

See: *Food Best for Human Consumption,* pp. 190 .

Energizing

Generate; place the coned fingers of one hand on lymphatic node, the other on the following acupressure locations:

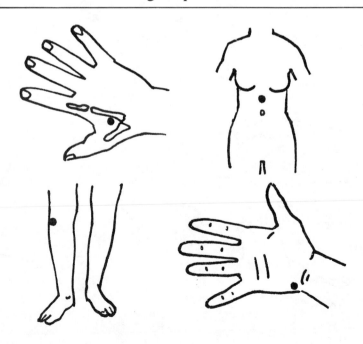

NIGHT SWEATS

Herbs

Sage.

Hops.

Yarrow,

Energizing

Generate; place the coned fingers of one hand on lymphatic node, the other on the following acupressure locations:

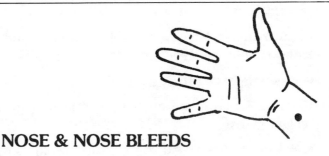

NOSE & NOSE BLEEDS

Herbs

Capsicum and hot water externally and internally.

Witch Hazel.

Horseradish - will help clear the nasal passages in nursing babies if allowed to breathe the fumes.

Vitamins

C, K.

Minerals

Calcium.

Diet

See: *Foods Best for Human Consumption* pp. 190 .

Energizing

Generate with arms above the head, then place the coned fingers of one hand on lymphatic node, the other on the following acupressure locations:

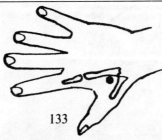

NURSING

(See: *Breasts, Lactation*).

OBESITY

Herbal Combinations

4-A Alfalfa, Comfrey, Horsetail Irish Moss, Lobelia, Oat Straw.

8-A Blessed Thistle, Capsicum, Ginger, Golden Seal, Gravel Root, Lobelia, Marshmallow, Parsley, Raspberry.

8-B Black Cohosh, Sarsaparilla, Ginseng, Licorice, False Unicorn, Blessed Thistle, Squawvine.

27-A Black Walnut, Chickweed, Dandelion, Echinacea, Fennel, Gotu Kola, Hawthorn, Licorice, Mandrake, Papaya, Safflowers.

29-A Capsicum, Irish Moss, Kelp, Parsley.

29-B Parsley, Watercress, Kelp, Irish Moss, Sarsaparilla, Black Walnut, Iceland Moss.

Chickweed plus herbal combination listed as number four above, — start slowly and work up to desired level.

Vitamins

B, C, E, Lecithin (two at each meal).

Minerals

Calcium, Magnesium, Potassium.

Diet

If your body is not too acid, drink lemon juice and distilled water - cut up ½ lemon and just put it in the water, start first thing in the morning, and keep adding water throughout the day. See: *Foods Best for Human Consumption*, and just stick as close to A1 as you can.

Energizing

Keep repeating, "Out big hips, in slim body" as you generate, jump and jog. Keep working up your time on the energizer without getting sore. When you get real hungry, generate; place the coned fingers of one hand on lymphatic node, the other on the following acupressure locations:

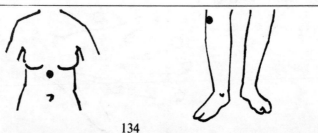

PAIN

Pain (See also: *Afterpain, Cramps, Headache, Migraine Headache*).

Herbal Combinations

1- Capsicum, Valerian Root, Wild Lettuce.

4-A Alfalfa, Comfrey, Horsetail, Irish Moss, Lobelia, Oat Straw.

14- Hops, Scullcap, Valerian Root.

Lobelia Extract.

Vitamins

B Complex in large doses, C, K.

Minerals

Calcium in large doses.

Diet

Lots of green, leafy vegetables. (See: *Correct Food Combinations*).

Energizing

Generate; place the coned fingers of one hand on lymphatic node, with the coned fingers of the other hand, pin point the exact area of the pain.

PALSY

Herbal Combinations

4-A   Alfalfa, Comfrey, Horsetail, Irish Moss, Lobelia, Oat Straw.

4-B   Black Cohosh, Capsicum, Ginger, Hops, Mistletoe, St. Johnswort, Valerian, Wood Betony.

14-   Hops, Scullcap, Valerian Root. (Take at night).

Vitamins

B Complex, E.

Minerals

Calcium.

Diet

See: *Correct Food Combinations,* pp. 189 .

Energizing

Generate; place the coned fingers of one hand on lymphatic node, the other on the following acupressure location:

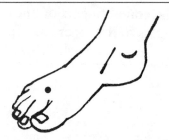

If you are unable to sit cross-legged, or bend to touch these places on your feet, have your partner touch each foot with coned fingers, while you cone your fingers on your lymphatic nodes.

Rest

A great deal of rest is needed.

PANCREAS

Herbal Combinations

3-A   Barberry, Burdock, Cascara Sagrada, Chaparral, Dandelion, Licorice, Red Clover, Sarsaparilla, Yarrow, Yellow Dock.

3-B   Red Clover, Chaparral, Licorice, Peach Bark, Oregon Grape, Stillingia, Cascarra Sagrada, Sarsaparilla, Prickly Ash Bark, Burdock, Buckthorn.

22-A   Angelica, Birch Leaves, Blessed Thistle, Chamomile, Dandelion, Gentian, Golden Rod, Horsetail, Liverwort Leaves, Lobelia, Parsley, Red Beet.

22-B   Barberry Bark, Cramp Bark, Fennel, Ginger, Catnip, Peppermint, Wild Yam.

23-B   Bistort, Blueberry Leaves, Buchu, Capsicum, Comfrey, Dandelion, Garlic, Golden Seal, Juniper Berries, Licorice, Marshmallow, Mullein, Uva-Ursi, Yarrow.

23-C   Juniper Berries, Uva-Ursi, Licorice, Mullein, Capsicum, Golden Seal Root.

Vitamins

A natural multi-vitamin.

Minerals

A natural multi-mineral.

Diet

See: *Hypoglycemic Diet* pp. 191 .

Enemas

Capsicum. (See also:*Enemas*).

Energizing

Generate; thinking generous thoughts, place the coned fingers of one hand on lymphatic node, the other on the following acupressure locations. Repeat, "The generous soul will be made fat, and the one freely watering others will be freely watered!" to the rhythm of the bounce.

(Illustrations next page...)

(Illustrations, Pancreas.)

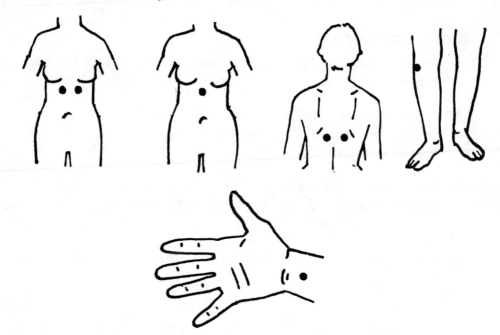

PARALYSIS

Herbal Combinations

6-A   Black Cohosh, Capsicum, Ginger, Hops, Mistletoe, St. Johnswort, Valerian, Wood Betony.

6-B   Black Cohosh, Capsicum, Hops, Mistletoe, Lobelia, Scullcap, Wood Betony, Lady's Slipper, Valerian.

14-   Hops, Scullcap, Valerian Root. (Take at night).

Oat Straw.

Scullcap.

Vitamins

B Complex, C.

Minerals

Iron, Phosphorous.

Diet

(See: *Correct Food Combinations,* also see: *Seven Day Cleanse*).

Energizing

Generate; place the coned fingers of one hand on lymphatic node, the other pin pointing troubled area, then proceed with the following acupressure locations:

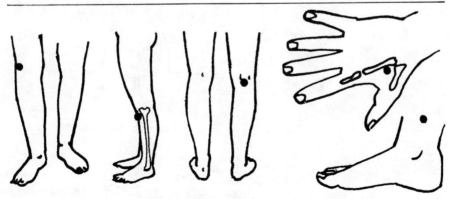

Note: If you cannot stand, you can sit on the machine or just place your feet on the machine and have your partner generate. Either of you can place coned fingers on the designated points.

PARASITES

Herbal Combinations

Black Walnut (2-6) all at once, one day, and Garlic (2-4).

28-B Cascara Sagrada, Comfrey, Culver's Root, Mandrake, Mullein, Pumpkin Seeds, Slippery Elm, Violet Leaves, Witch Hazel.

Take (2-6) of the above combination the next day. Continue this routine for two weeks, then skip a day between each combination for the next two weeks. If your family is around pets, you should do this routine twice a year. Your children will be much calmer.

Enemas

Garlic. (See: *Enemas*).

Energizing

Generate; place the coned fingers of one hand on the lymphatic node, place the other hand flat on the abdomen. Proceed with *stroking* motion in the direction of the arrows in the region of the large intestine.

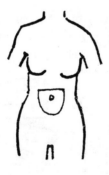 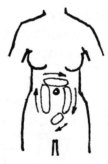

PARATHYROID

(See Anxiety);

PARKINSON'S DISEASE

(See also: *Palsy*).

Herbal Combinations

19-A Alfalfa, Dandelion, Kelp.

19-B Yellow Dock, Red Beet, Nettle, Burdock, Strawberry Leaves, Mullein, Lobelia.

32   Capsicum, Chickweed, Damiana, Echinacea, Garlic, Ginseng, Gotu Kola, Periwinkle, Sarsaparilla, Saw Palmetto.

Ginseng.

Vitamins

A, B, C, E, a natural muti-vitamin, lecithin.

Minerals

Calcium, Magnesium, a natural muti-mineral.

Diet

See: *Correct Food Combinations* pp 189 .

Enemas

Cleansing - very important. (See also: *Enemas*).

Energizing

Generate; place the coned fingers of one hand on lymphatic node, the other on the following acupressure location, then continue pin pointing wherever face, neck, or body limbs feel rigid.

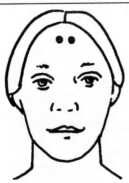

PERSPIRATION

Herbs

Excessive:
Wood Betony.

For Odor:
Horsetail (foot bath). Liquid Chlorophyll.

To Produce Perspiration:
Ginger (bath). Yarrow, Hyssop.

Diet

See: *Correct Food Combinations.*

Energizing

Generate; place the coned fingers of one hand on lymphatic node, the other on the following acupressure location:

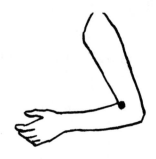

PHLEBITIS
(Inflammation of a vein).

Herbal Combinations

16-A Capsicum, Echinacea, Myrrh, Yarrow.

16-B Capsicum, Echinacea, Golden Seal, Yarrow.

Comfrey packs or poultices.

Vitamins

C, E, Lecithin.

Minerals

Calcium, Iron.

Diet

See: *Correct Food Combinations.*

Energizing

Generate; place the coned fingers of one hand on lymphatic node, the other on the following acupressure location, then continue pin pointing the distressed area. CAUTION: If blood clots are present, DO NOT use the machine.

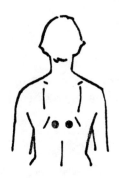

PINEAL GLAND

Energizing

Generate; place the coned fingers of one hand on lymphatic node, the other on the following acupressure location. Then repeat: "I will become more friendly, I will speak to God, I will speak to my husband (wife), I will speak with my neighbor," etc., to the rhythm of the bounce.

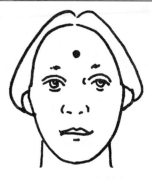

PINK EYE or CONJUNCTIVITIS
(See also: *Eyes*).

Herbal Combinations

7 A&B Bayberry, Eyebright, Golden Seal.

Capsicum (optional). See also: *Eye Wash*.

Generate; place the coned fingers of one hand on lymphatic node, the other on the following acupressure location, then continue pin pointing the eye area.

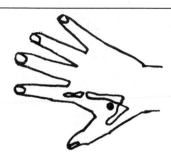

PILES
(See: *Hemorrhoids and Piles*).

PITUITARY GLAND

Herbal Combinations

12-A Capsicum, Ginseng, Gotu Kola.

3-A Alfalfa, Dandelion, Kelp.

19-B Yellow Dock, Red Beet, Nettle, Burdock, Strawberry Leaves, Mullein, Lobelia.

29-A Capsicum, Irish Moss, Kelp, Parsley.

29-B Parsley, Watercress, Kelp, Irish Moss, Sarsaparilla, Black Walnut, Iceland Moss.

Vitamins

C, E, Lecithin.

Minerals

A natural multi-mineral.

Diet

See: *Correct Food Combinations.*

Energizing

Refer to Gland Chart, pp. 203 . Generate, place the coned fingers of one hand on lymphatic node, and the coned hands of the other on area # 1. Then place coned fingers on area # 2, continue with the following acupressure location. Repeat, "I feel healthy, I feel happy, I feel terrific!" to the rhythm of the bounce.

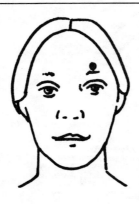

PLEURISY

(See also: *Lungs, Pneumonia*).

Herbs

Poultice - ½ t. Capsicum, 1 Tblsp. Lobelia, 3 Tblsp. Slippery Elm. Mix with mineral water. Leave on chest only 1 hour. Dispose of (See also: *Poultice*).

Lobelia.

Mullein.

Slippery Elm.

Vitamins

A, C, E.

Minerals

Calcium.

Diet

Lots of water and juices.

Energizing

Generate; place the coned fingers of one hand on lymphatic node, the other on the following acupressure locations:

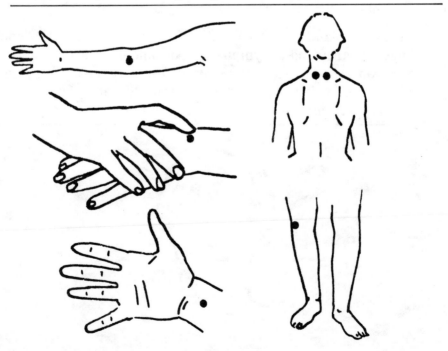

PNEUMONIA

(See also: *Lungs*).

Herbal Combinations

16-A Capsicum, Echinacea, Myrrh, Yarrow.

16-B Capsicum, Echinacea, Golden Seal, Yarrow.

16-C Plantain, Black Walnut, Golden Seal Root, Bugleweed, Marshmallow, Lobelia.

21-A Comfrey, Lobelia, Marshmallow, Mullein, Slippery Elm.

21-B Marshmallow, Mullein, Comfrey, Lobelia, Chickweed.

Lobelia.

Mullein.

Vitamins

A, C, E.

Minerals

Calcium.

Poultices

4 capsules Lobelia, 1 capsule Quinine, 1 t. oil of Turpentine. Mix with Vaseline or Vicks. Put on cloth on chest. (See also: *Muastard Plaster.*).

Enemas

Cleansing. (See: *Enema*).

Diet

Drink as much juice and water as possible. Stay away from milk products.

Energizing

If unable to get out of bed, place feet on machine. Partner will generate; either person may place coned fingers of both hands on chest area, then continue with the following acupressure locations:

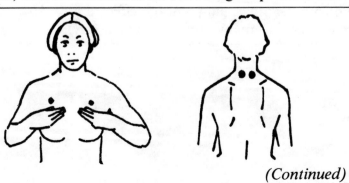

(Continued)

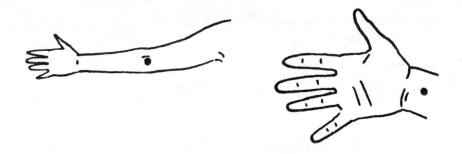

POISON IVY & OAK

Herbal Combinations

3-A   Barberry, Burdock, Cascara Sagrada, Chaparral, Dandelion, Licorice, Red Clover, Sarsaparilla, Yarrow, Yellow Dock.

3-B   Red Clover, Chaparral, Licorice, Peach Bark, Oregon Grape, Stillingia, Cascara Sagrada, Sarsaparilla, Prickly Ash Bark, Burdock, Buckthorn.

Aloe Vera, internally and externally.

Burdock.

Vitamins

C, high doses.

Diet

Water and juice.

Enemas

Cleansing (See: *Enemas*).

Energizing

Generate; place the coned fingers of one hand on lymphatic node, and with the other, pin point the affected area. Use machine for a short time, but many times during the day.

POT BELLY

Herbal Combinations

27- Black Walnut, Chickweed, Dandelion, Echinacea, Fennel, Gotu Kola, Hawthorn, Licorice, Mandrake, Papaya, Safflowers.

Vitamins

A natural multi-vitamin.

Minerals

A natural multi-mineral.

Enemas

Cleansing - often. (See also: *Enemas*).

Diet

No meats, cheese, sugar, or salt until the pot belly is gone.

Energizing

Generate; place the coned fingers of one hand on the lymphatic node, place the entire hand over the pot belly. Then continue with coned fingers on the following acupressure points:

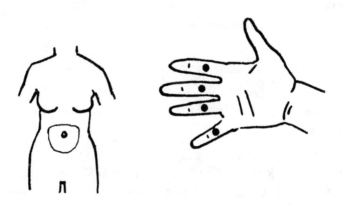

PREGNANCY
(See also: *Afterbirth, Birth Defects, Childbirth*).

Herbal Combinations

4-A   Alfalfa, Comfrey, Horsetail, Irish Moss, Lobelia, Oat Straw

8-A   Blessed Thistle, Capsicum, Ginger, Golden Seal, Gravel Root, Lobelia, Marshmallow, Parsley, Raspberry.

8-B   Black Cohosh, Sarsaparilla, Ginseng, Licorice, False Unicorn, Blessed Thistle, Squawvine.

33-A   Black Cohosh, Lobelia, Pennyroyal, Raspberry, Squawvine.

33-B   Squawvine, Blessed Thistle, Black Cohosh, Pennyroyal, False Unicorn, Red Raspberry, Lobelia.

Use the last two herbal combinations listed above only at the *end* of pregnancy.

Raspberry.

For complications: Lobelia.

DO NOT use the following herbs during early pregnancy: Pennyroyal, Rue.

Vitamins

B, E, a natural multi-vitamin.

Minerals

Manganese, a natural multi-mineral.

Diet

See: *Correct Food Combinations*. Try to keep your calories down.

Energizing

Start with walking in place or shuffling feet on the machine. Progress: kicking legs out in front, to side, to back, and generate. See your doctor before doing vigorous exercise, unless you were used to it before becoming pregnant.

NOTE: DO NOT stimulate the following point during pregnancy, it may start your labor.

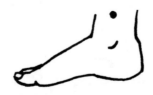

PROSTATE

Herbal Combinations

26-A Black Cohosh, Capsicum, Ginger, Golden Seal, Gotu Kola, Kelp, Licorice, Lobelia.

26-B Capsicum, Uva-Ursi, Parsley, Golden Seal Root, Gravel Root, Juniper Berry, Marshmallow, Ginger, Ginseng.

28-B Cascara Sagrada, Comfrey, Culver's Root, Mandrake, Mullein, Pumpkin Seeds, Slippery Elm, Violet Leaves, Witch Hazel.

Vitamins

B, C, E.

Minerals

Zinc, Manganese.

Enemas

Cleansing, very important. (See *Enemas*).

Diet

See: *Correct Food Combinations,* and *Food Best for Human Consumption.*

Energizing

Generate; place the coned fingers of one hand on lymphatic node, the other on the following acupressure locations:

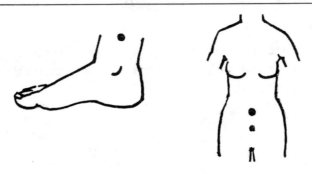

PSORIASIS

Herbal Combinations

3-A Barberry, Burdock, Cascara Sagrada, Chaparral, Dandelion, Licorice, Red Clover, Sarsaparilla, Yarrow, Yellow Dock.

3-B Red Clover, Chaparral, Licorice, Peach Bark, Oregon Grape, Stillingia, Cascara Sagrada, Sarsaparilla, Prickly Ash Bark, Burdock, Buckthorn.

4-A Alfalfa, Comfrey, Irish Moss, Lobelia, Oat Straw.

4-B Horsetail, Comfrey, Oat Straw, Lobelia.

Burdock.

Aloe Vera - internally and externally.

Jojoba oil - externally.

Vitamins

A, B, C, E, Lecithin.

Minerals

Calcium, Magnesium.

Enemas

Cleansing (See: *Enemas*).

Diet

Eat lots of dark green, leafy vegetables. (See: *Correct Food Combinations,* and *Food Best for Human Consumption*).

Energizer

Generate; place the coned fingers of one hand on lymphatic node, use the other to pin point the area, then continue on the following acupressure location:

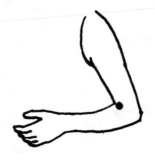

PYORRHEA
(See also: *Mouth Sores*)

Herbal Combinations

30-A Capsicum, Golden Seal, Myrrh.

Golden Seal.

Aloe Vera - internally and externally.

Vitamin

A, B, C, E. (Large doses of C).

Mineral

Calcium and Phosphorous.

Diet

Stay away from acid-forming foods; tomatoes, citrus, etc.

Energizing

Generate; place the coned fingers of one hand on lymphatic node, and with the other, pin point the gum area.

REJECTION
(See Pancreas)

REPRODUCTION
(See: *Sex*).

RESPIRATION
(See: *Lungs*).

RHEUMATIC FEVER
(See also: *Fever, Joints*).

Herbal Combinations

13-A Capsicum, Garlic, Hawthorn.

3-B Capsicum, Parsley, Ginger, Garlic, Ginseng, Golden Seal Root.

16-A Capsicum, Echinacea, Myrrh, Yarrow.

16-B Capsicum, Echinacea, Golden Seal, Yarrow.

22-A Angelica, Birch Leaves, Blessed Thistle, Chamomile, Dandelion, Gentian, Golden Rod, Horsetail, Liverwort Leaves, Lobelia, Parsley, Red Beet.

22-B Barberry Bark, Cramp Bark, Fennel, Ginger, Catnip, Peppermint, Wild Yam.

Lobelia.

Vitamins

A, B, C, E, P, PABA.

Minerals

Calcium, Zinc.

Enema

Cleansing (See: *Enemas*).

Diet

Eat lots of vegetables and fruit. (See: *Correct Food Combinations*).

Energizing

Generate many times per day, but for short periods of time. Place coned fingers of both hands on lymphayic nodes. Slowly change hands from one sore joint to another. Breathe in through the nose, and out through the mouth, think positively about new health coming in and pain and disease going out. Repeat: "In new health, out pain and disease!" to the rhythm of the bounce. If heart is affected see also: *Heart*.

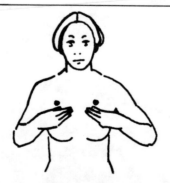

RHEUMATISM
(See also: *Arthritis, Gout*).

Herbal Combinations

1- Capsicum, Valerian Root, Wild Lettuce.

2- Alfalfa, Black Cohosh, Bromalain Powder, Burdock Root, Capsicum, Centaury, Chaparral, Comfrey, Lobelia, Yarrow, Yucca.

3-A Alfalfa, Comfrey, Horsetail, Irish Moss, Lobelia, Oat Straw.

24-A Aloe Vera, Comfrey, Golden Seal, Slippery Elm.

24-B Comfrey, White Oah Bark, Mullein, Black Walnut, Marshmallow, Gravel Root, Wormwood, Lobelia, Scullcap.

Alfalfa.

Yucca.

Vitamins

B, C, E, P, F.

Minerals

Calcium, Potassium, Magnesium.

Enemas

Cleansing (See: *Enemas*).

Diet

No red meat. Whole rice instead of potatoes. All the vegetables you can eat or vegetable juice. No sweets.

Energizing

Necessary to keep body in balance. Start generating with coned fingers on lymphatic nodes, then with one coned hand at base of skull and the other at the end of tailbone. Always breathe deeply, in through the nose, and out through the mouth. Start first thing in the morning, then at any time during the day after you have sat or lain down. Must keep moving even if it hurts. A few weeks of this schedule, and thinking positively, and you will feel less and less pain. Don't quit or it will come back.

(Continued)

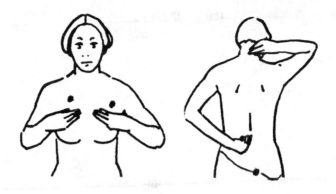

RIBS
(See also: *Bones*).

Energizing

Generate; place coned fingers of one hand on lymphatic node, place the other pin pointing painful area. Then place coned fingers on the following acupressure location:

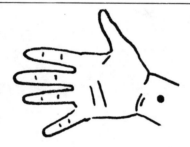

RICKETS AND OSTEOMALACIA
(See: *Bones*).

Energizing

Generate; place the coned fingers of one hand on lymphatic node, the other pin pointing painful area. Then place coned fingers on the following acupressure location:

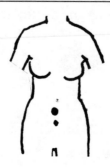

RINGWORM

Herbal Combinations

3-A Barberry, Burdock, Cacars Sagrada, Chaparral, Dandelion, Licorice, Red Clover, Sarsaparilla, Yarrow, Yellow Dock.

Black Walnut and Garlic every other day. Herbal Pumpkin the other days, for two weeks.

Black Walnut Extract or Apple Cider on the skin.

Enemas

Garlic. (See: *Enemas*).

Diet

No sweets at all.

Energizing

Generate with coned fingers on lymphatic nodes in chest or groin area. (See Lymph Chart).

SCALDS
(See: *Burns*).

SCARLET FEVER

Herbs

Red Raspberry	Yellow Dock	Bayberry Tea
Red Clover	Desert Tea	Myrrh
		Golden Seal

Packs

See: *Mumps*.

Vitamins

High doses of C.

Minerals

Calcium.

Enemas

Lobelia, Bayberry, Catnip and Garlic. (See: *Enemas*).

Diet

Juices, pure water, raw foods blended in a blender.

Energizing

When able, generate, with coned fingers in the chest or groin area. (See Lymph Chart).

SCIATICA
(See: *Arthritis, Gout, Rheumatism*).

Energizing

Generate; place coned fingers on the dimples of your buttocks. Then continue placing the coned fingers of one hand on lymphatic node, the other on the following acupressure locations:

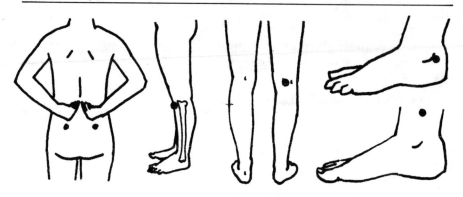

SEA SICKNESS
(See: *Motion Sickness*).

SENILITY
(See: *Age Spots, Vitality*).

SEX DESIRE

(See: *Frigidity, Sterility*).

Herbal Combinations

To Decrease:

14- Hops, Scullcap, Valerian Root.

To Increase, Impotency, or Premature Ejaculation:

32- Capsicum, Chickweed, Damiana, Echinacea, Garlic, Ginseng, Gotu Kola, Periwinkle, Sarsaparilla, Saw Palmetto.

Vitamins

E.

Minerals

Zinc.

Energizing

Generate; place the coned fingers of one hand on lympahtic node, and the other on the following acupressure locations:

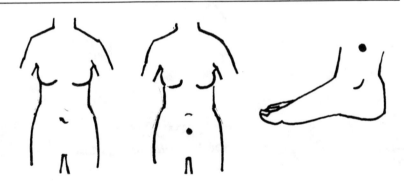

SHINGLES

Herbal Combinations

19-A   Alfalfa, Dandelion, Kelp.

Vitamins

B Complex, E oil directly on blisters.

Minerals

Calcium, Zinc.

Energizing

Generate; place the coned fingers of one hand on lymphatic node, the other on the following acupressure locations:

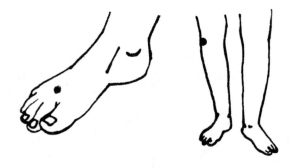

SHOCK
(See also: *Fainting and Anxiety*).

SHOULDER

Energizing

Generate; place the coned fingers of one hand on lymphatic node. place the other on the following acupressure location. Also *stroke* the pained area. NOTE: it is more feasible to work with a partner.

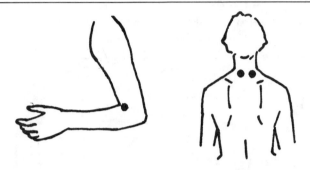

SINUS
(See also: *Mucous Membrane*).

Energizing

Generate; place the coned fingers of hand on lymphatic node, place the other pin pointing the painful sinus area. Then continue placing coned fingers on the following acupressure locations:

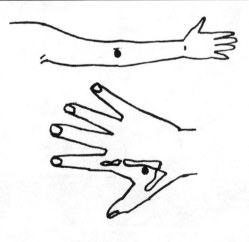

SKIN DISEASE
(See also: *Acne, Eczema, Psoriasis,* etc.)

Energizing

Generate; place the coned fingers of one hand on lymphatic node, place the other on the following acupressure locations: Repeat, "I will live in harmony with God's laws, I will live in harmony with my mother, I will live in harmony with my father, I will live in harmony with my husband (wife), I will live in harmony with my neighbor," etc., in rhythm with the bounce.

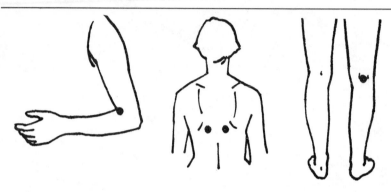

SLEEP
(See: *Insomnia*).

SMOKING
(See also: *Cough* and *Seven Day Cleanse).*

Herbal Combinations

To decrease desire and support the nervous system.

3-A   Barberry, Burdock, Cascara Sagrada, Chaparral, Dandelion, Licorice, Red Clover, Sarsaparilla, Yarrow, Yellow Dock.

21-A   Comfrey, Lobelia, Marshmallow, Mullein, Slippery Elm.

14-   Hops, Scullcap, Valerian Root, plus take extra Slippery Elm.

Vitamins

C - large doses.

Minerals

Calcium.

Energizing

Generate; very important to take deep breaths as if you were inhaling - in through the mouth and out through the nose. As you inhale, throw arms up and out away from body, as you exhale, cross arms over chest. Do this several times. Then continue placing both hands with coned fingers on lymphatic nodes in chest area. (See Lymph Chart). Then place the coned fingers of one hand on lymphatic node, place the other on the following acupressure location:

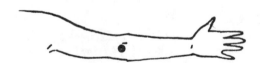

SNEEZING

Energizing

Generate; place the coned fingers of one hand on lymphatic node, the other on the following acupressure location:

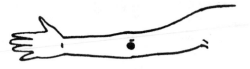

SORES
(See: *Wounds*).

SORE THROAT
(*See Throat*).

SPLEEN

Herbal Combinations

3-A   Barberry, Burdock, Cascara Sagrada, Chaparral, Dandelion, Licorice, Red Clover, Sarsaparilla, Yarrow, Yellow Dock.

3-B   Red Clover, Chaparral, Licorice, Poke Root, Peach Bark, Oregon Grape, Stillingia, Cascara Sagrada, Sarsaparilla, Prickly Ash Bark, Burdock, Buckthorn.

22-A   Angelica, Birch Leaves, Blessed Thistle, Chamomile, Dandelion, Gentian, Golden Rod, Horsetail, Liverwort Leaves, Lobelia, Parsley, Red Beet.

22-B   Barberry Bark, Cramp Bark, Fennel, Ginger, Catnip, Peppermint, Wild Yam.

Vitamins

C - large doses.

Minerals

A natural multi-vitamin.

Enemas

Capsicum. (See: *Enemas*).

Diet

See: *Correct Food Combinations*.

Energizing

Generate; place the coned fingers of one hand on lymphatic node, place the other on the following acupressure locations: Repeat, "I feel healthy, I feel happy, I feel cheerful, I feel festive!" to the rhythm of the bounce.

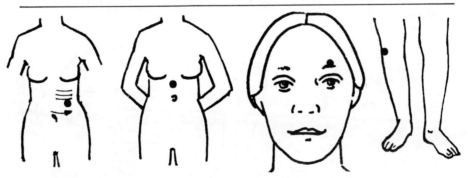

SPRAINS
(See *Inflammation*).

STERILITY
(See: *Frigidity*).

STOMACH
(See also: *Ulcers, Gastritis*).

Herbal Combinations

4-A Alfalfa, Comfrey, Horsetail, Irish Moss, Lobelia, Oat Straw.

17- Fennel, Wild Yam, Peppermint, Ginger, Papaya, Spearmint, Catnip, Lobelia.

30-A Capsicum, Golden Seal, Myrrh.

30-B Marshmallow, Slippery Elm, Comfrey, Lobelia, Ginger, Wild Yam.

Vitamins

A natural multi-vitamin.

Minerals

Mineral water, a natural multi-mineral.

Diet

Keep a diary on what is upsetting the stomach, and what hurts the mouth. DO NOT eat these foods again until the stomach is healed.

Enemas

Cleansing. (See *Enemas*).

Energizing

Generate; place the coned fingers of one hand on lymphatic node, place the other on the following acupressure locations and repeat: "God is faithful to me, and cannot lie to me!" to the rhythm of the bounce.

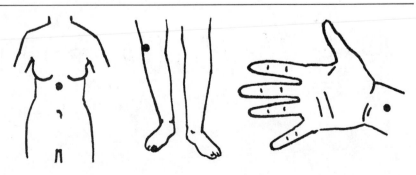

STONES
(See: *Gall Bladder, Kidney*).

STRESS
(See: *Nerves*).

ST. VITUS DANCE
(See: *Nerves*).

STROKE
(See also: *High Blood Pressure* and *Paralysis*).

Herbal Combinations

(*For Paralysis*).

12-A Capsicum and Garlic, (3) Oil of Garlic capsules, (1) capsule: Capsicum, Ginseng, Gotu Kola, plus extra Gotu Kola, (1) capsule:

27- Black Walnut, Chickweed, Dandelion, Echinacea, Fennel, Gotu Kola, Hawthorn, Licorice, Mandrake, Papaya, Safflowers, and (1) Grape Vine.

Vitamins

A natural multi-vitamin.

Minerals

A natural multi-mineral.

Diet

See: *Correct Food Combinations.*

Enemas

Cleansing or Garlic (See also: *Enemas*).

Energizing

Generate; with or without partner, place coned fingers of one hand on lymphatic node, place other on the following acupressure locations:

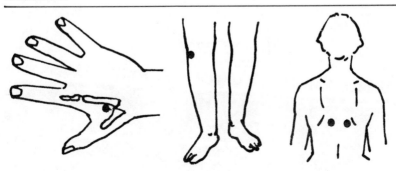

STY
(See also: *Blood Purifier, Infection*).

Herbs

Sty must be opened , and a hot, moist poultice of strong Sarsaparilla Tea should be applied over the eye.

Generate; place the coned fingers of one hand on lymphatic node, the other pin pointing sty.

SUNBURN
(See: *Burns*).

SUN STROKE

Herbs

Pennyroyal.

Vitamins

B, C, E.

Minerals

Sodium.

Energizing

Generate; if the person cannot stand, place his feet on the machine, either person place one hand with coned fingers on lymphatic node, place the other hand with coned fingers on the following acupressure location.

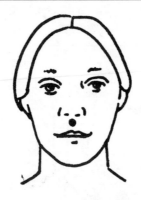

SWEATS
(See: *Night Sweats*).

SWELLING
(See: *Inflammation and Swelling*).

SYPHILIS
(See: *Venereal Disease*).

TEETH

Herbal Combinations

For Toothache or Decayed Teeth:
4-A   Alfalfa, Comfrey, Horsetail, Irish Moss, Lobelia, Oat Straw.

For Toothache:
1-   Capsicum, Valerian Root, Wild Lettuce.

For Loose Teeth or Toothache:

24-A   Aloe Vera, Comfrey, Golden Seal, Slippery Elm.

Vitamins

A, B, C, D.

Minerals

Calcium, Magnesium, Phosphorus, Iodine.

Diet

See: *Food Best for Human Consumption.*

Energizing

Generate; place the coned fingers of one hand on lymphatic node, place the other pin pointing pain in tooth. Then continue with coned fingers on the following acupressure location:

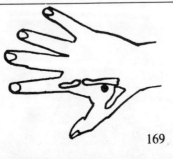

169

TETANUS

Herbs
Capsicum.

Lobelia Extract.

Vitamins
C, high doses.

Energizing
Generate; place the coned fingers of one hand on lymphatic node, place the other on the following acupressure locations:

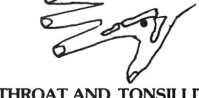

THROAT AND TONSILLITIS

Herbal Combinations
20-A   Barberry, Buckthorn, Cascara Sagrada, Capsicum, Couch Grass, Ginger, Licorice, Lobelia, Red Clover.

For Tonsillitis:

5-A   Capsicum, Chamomile, Golden Seal, Lemon Grass, Myrrh, Peppermint, Rose Hips, Sage, Slippery Elm, Yarrow.

Sore Throat and Tonsillitis:

16-A   Capsicum, Echinacea, Myrrh, Yarrow.

16-B   Capsicum, Echinacea, Golden Seal, Yarrow.

Vitamins
A, C, E, Pantothenic Acid.

Minerals
Calcium.

Enemas
Garlic (See: *Enemas*).

(Continued)

(Continued from previous page).

Diet

Juices and pure water.

Energizing

Generate; place the coned fingers of one hand on lymphatic node, place the other on the following acupressure locations:

Throat: *Tonsillitis:*

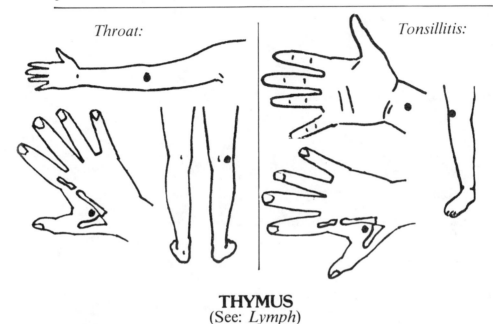

THYMUS
(See: *Lymph*)

Energizing

Generate; place both hands with coned fingers on the thymus nodes, (See Lymph Chart). Repeat: "I am enthusiastic, I am interested in life, I am interested in my family, I am interested in my projects, I feel calmness within myself, I feel calmness with others!" to the rhythm of the bounce.

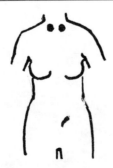

THYROID

Herbal Combinations

29-A Capsicum, Irish Moss, Kelp, Parsley.

29-B Parsley, Watercress, Kelp, Irish Moss, Sarsaparilla, Black Walnut, Iceland Moss.

Low:
30-A Bayberry, Golden Seal, Myrrh.

Vitamins

C, E.

Minerals

Iodine.

Diet

See: *Correct Food Combinations.*

Energizing

Generate; place the coned fingers of one hand on lymphatic node, place the other on the following acupressure locations: Repeat, "I feel goodness, I feel pleasantness, I feel kindness!" to the rhythm of the bounce.

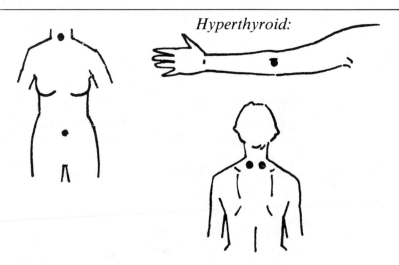

Hyperthyroid:

TICS
(See also: *Nerves*).

Energizing

Generate; place the coned fingers of one hand on lymphatic node, the other on the following acupressure locations:

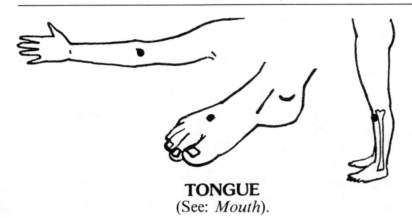

TONGUE
(See: *Mouth*).

TONSILLITIS
(See: *Throat*).

TOOTHACHE
(See: *Teeth*).

TRACHEA
(See also: *Respiration*).

Energizing

Generate; place the coned fingers of one hand on lymphatic node, the other on the following acupressure locations:

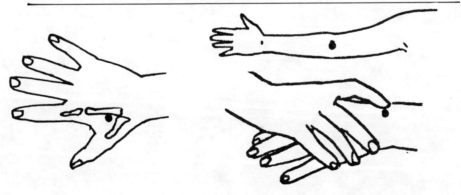

TROUBLED
(See Thymus)

TUBERCULOSIS
(See: *Lungs*).

TUMORS
(See also: *Cancer*).

Herbal Combinations

4-A Alfalfa, Comfrey, Horsetail, Irish Moss, Lobelia, Oat Straw.

28-A Barberry, Black Walnut, Catnip, Chickweed, Comfrey, Cyani Flowers, Dandelion, Echinacea, Fenugreek, Gentian, Golden Seal, Irish Moss, Mandrake, Myrrh Gum, Pink Root, Poke Root, Safflowers, St. Johnswort, Yellow Dock.

28-B Cascara Sagrada, Comfrey, Culver's Root, Mandrake, Mullein, Pumpkin Seeds, Slippery Elm, Violet Leaves, Witch Hazel.

NOTE: Take Combination # 2 listed above one day, and combination # 3 listed above the next day.

Energizing

Generate; place the coned fingers of one hand on lymphatic node, place the other pin pointing tumor.

ULCERS
(See also: *Stomach*).

Herbal Combinations

4-A   Alfalfa, Comfrey, Horsetail, Irish Moss, Lobelia, Oat Straw.

24-A   Aloe Vera, Comfrey, Golden Seal, Sippery Elm.

30-A   Capsicum, Golden Seal, Myrrh.

30-B   Marshmallow, Slippery Elm, Comfrey, Lobelia, Ginger, Wild Yam.

Vitamins

B, C, E.

Minerals

Calcium.

Diet

Drink Slippery Elm Tea or Aloe Vera before you eat anything. Eat low fiber, bland foods.

Enemas

Slippery Elm (See: *Enemas*).

Energizing

Generate; plave the coned fingers of one hand on lymphatic node, the other on the following acupressure locations:

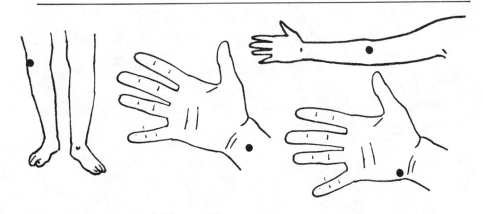

Leg Ulcers
(See: *Wounds*).

UNAPPRECIATED   *(See Intestines - Small)*
UNCOMMUNICATIVE   *(See Pineal)*

UNCONSCOUSNESS
(See: *Fainting*).

UNDESIREABLE   *(See Hypothalamus)*

UNHAPPY
(See: *Spleen or Pituitary*).

UNSUPPORTIVE   *(See Ear)*

URINATION
(See also: *Bladder, Kidneys*).

Herbal Combinations

Bloody:
Marshmallow, White Oak Bark, Comfrey.

Difficulty:
St. Johnswort, Slippery Elm.

To Increase:
18-A   Chamomile, Dandelion, Juniper, Parsley, Uva-Ursi.
Urethral Irritation:
35-   Squawvine, Chick weed, Slippery Elm, Comfrey, Yellow Dock, Golden Seal Root, Mullein, Marshmallow.

Vitamins

A, C, E.

Minerals

Calcium, Zinc.

Diet

Eat substantial amounts of carrots, dark green, leafy vegetables, and fruit.

Energizing

Generate; place the coned fingers of one hand on lymphatic node, the other on the following acupressure locations:

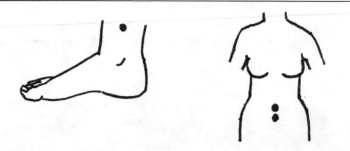

UTERUS

Herbs

Dong Quai.

Herbal Combinations

8-A Blessed Thistle, Capsicum, Ginger, Golden Seal, Gravel Root, Lobelia, Marshmallow, Parsley, Raspberry.

8-B Black Cohosh, Sarsaparilla, Ginseng, Licorice, False Unicorn, Blessed Thistle, Squawvine.

Douche:

35- Squawvine, Chickweed, Slippery Elm, Comfrey, Yellow Dock, Golden Seal Root, Mullein, Marshmallow.

Vitamins

E.

Minerals

Calcium.

Diet

See: *Food Best for Human Consumption.*

Energizing

Generate; place the coned fingers of one hand on lymphatic node, and the other hand on the following acupressure locations:

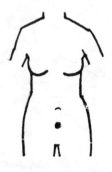
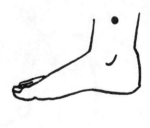

VAGINA

Herbal Combinations

8-A   Blessed Thistle, Capsicum, Ginger, Golden Seal, Gravel Root, Lobelia, Marshmallow, Parsley, Raspberry.

8-B   Black Cohosh, Sarsaparilla, Ginseng, Licorice, False Unicorn, Blessed Thistle, Squawvine.

35-   *Douche* (See also: *Douche*).
Squawvine, Chickweed, Slippery Elm, Comfrey, Yellow Dock, Golden Seal Root, Mullein, Marshmallow.

Mineral Water.

Vitamins

A, C, E.

Minerals

Calcium, Zinc.

Diet

See: *Food Best for Human Consumption.*

Energizing

Generate; place the coned fingers of one hand on lymphatic node, the other on the following acupressure locations:

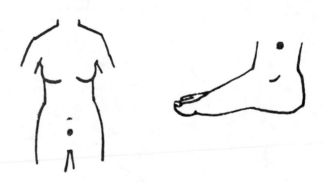

VARICOSE VEINS
(See also: *Circulation*).

Herbal Combinations

4-A Alfalfa, Comfrey, Horsetail, Irish Moss, Lobelia, Oat Straw.

4-B Horsetail, Comfrey, Oat Straw, Lobelia.

13-A Capsicum, Garlic, Hawthorn.

Capsicum, Parsley, Ginger, Garlic, Ginseng.

13-B Capsicum, Parsley, Ginger, Garlic, Ginseng, Golden Seal Root.

White Oak Bark.

Vitamins

C, E, Lecithin.

Minerals

Calcium.

Packs

White Oak Bark.

Diet

See: *Food Best for Human Consumption.*

Energizing

Generate: place coned fingers of both hands on lymphatic nodes in chest area. Partner place his coned fingers on the following acupressure location:

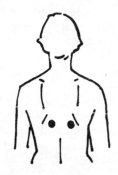

VENEREAL DISEASES

Herbal Combinations

3-A Barberry, Burdock, Cascara Sagrada, Chaparral, Dandelion, Licorice, Red Clover, Sarsaparilla, Yarrow, Yellow Dock.

Douches (See also: *Douche*).

35- Squawvine, Chickweed, Slippery Elm, Comfrey, Yellow Dock, Golden Seal Root, Mullein, Marshmallow.

Vitamins

A, B, C, E, K.

Minerals

Calcium, Magnesium, Zinc.

Diet

Cleanse (See *Seven Day Cleanse*).

Energizing

Generate; place the coned fingers of both hands on lymphatic nodes in chest or groin area, then *strength bounce* with both feet off machine with fingers remaining in same areas. Pin point # 45 of Gland Chart. (See: Gland Chart).

VERTIGO
(See also: *Heart, Blood Pressure*).

Energizing

Generate; place the coned fingers of one hand on lymphatic node, the other on the following acupressure locations:

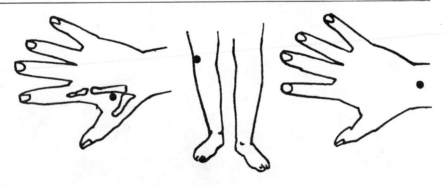

VITALITY
(See: *Endurance, Energy*).

VOICE
(See: *Hoarseness*).

VOMITING
(See also: *Morning Sickness, Nausea*).

Energizing

Generate; place the coned fingers of one hand on lymphatic node, the other on the following acupressure locations:

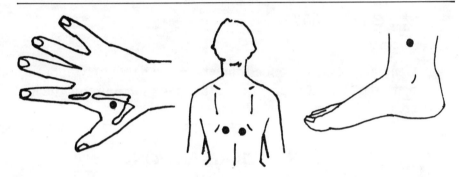

WARTS

Herbs

Milkweed - externally.

Buckthorn.

Vitamins

E, Castor Oil - externally.

A, C, E - internally.

Minerals

A vegetable multi-mineral.

Diet

See: *Correct Food Combinations.*

Energizing

Generate; plave the coned fingers of one hand on lymphatic node, place the coned fingers of the other hand pin pointing the irritated area.

WATER RETENTION

Herbal Combinations

4-A   Alfalfa, Comfrey, Horsetail, Irish Moss, Lobelia, Oat Straw.

18-A   Chamomile, Dandelion, Juniper, Parsley, Uva-Ursi.

19-A   Alfalfa, Dandelion, Kelp.

Vitamins

B, C.

Minerals

Calcium, Potassium.

Diet

Eat substantial amounts of dark green, leafy vegetables and fruit.

Energizing

Generate; place the coned fingers of both hands on the lymphatic nodes.

WEARY

(See: *Bladder*).

WITTS END

(See Intestines - Sigmoid Colon)

WHOOPING COUGH

(See also: *Cough*).

Herbs

Ginseng, Mullein, Thyme.

Vitamins

C.

Minerals

Calcium.

Diet

Juices, fruits and vegetables.

Energizing

Generate; place coned fingers and rest of fingers spread across chest area. If small baby, hold him in your arms and generate or lay him on the machine and generate it with your foot.

WORMS

(See: *Parasites*).

WORRY

(See: *Sex Desire*)

WOUNDS

Herbal Combinations

3-A Barberry, Burdock, Cascara Sagrada, Chaparral, Dandelion, Licorice, Red Clover, Sarsaparilla, Yarrow, Yellow Dock.

4-A Alfalfa, Comfrey, Horsetail, Irish Moss, Lobelia, Oat Straw.

24-A Aloe Vera, Comfrey, Golden Seal, Slippery Elm.

24-B Comfrey, White Oak Bark, Mullein, Black Walnut, Marshmallow, Gravel Root, Wormwood, Lobelia, Scullcap.

30-A Capsicum, Golden Seal, Myrrh.

Aloe Vera.

Poultices

Use above herbs.

Vitamins

A, B, C, E.

Minerals

Calcium, Zinc.

Diet

Wheat germ, fruits and vegetables.

Energizing

Generate; place the coned fingers of one hand on lymphatic node, place other coned fingers pin pointing wound.

WRIST PAIN

Energizing

Generate; place the coned fingers of one hand on lymphatic node, the other on the followiong acupressure locations:

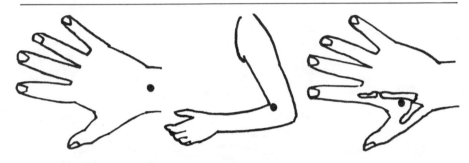

YEAST INFECTION

Herbal Combinations

35- Squawvine, Chickweed, Slippery Elm, Comfrey, Yellow Dock, Golden Seal Root, Mullein, Marshmallow.

Douche

Use above herbs (See also: *Douche*).

Vitamin

A, C, E, Acidophilus.

Mineral

Calcium.

Diet

Absolutely no sweets, coffee, or alcohol. (See also: *Food Best for Human Consumption*).

Energizing

Generate; place the coned fingers of one hand on lymphatic node, place the other on # 45 of gland chart. (See: *Gland Chart*).

YOUTHFULNESS
(See: *Thymus*).

SECTION TWO
Special Diets & Recipes

STEPS TO HEALTH—DURING AND AFTER COLON THERAPY

ALWAYS start at the bottom step and work your way up. Go slowly and steadily as your body heals. Try no to take 2 steps at a time - you may find yourself at the very beginning again.

EVERY DAY: Drink at least 6 glasses of water, 3 upon arising. Try to drink a gallon (16) glasses. If you feel bloated drink warm water. TAKE ACIDOPHILUS NIGHT & MORNING!!

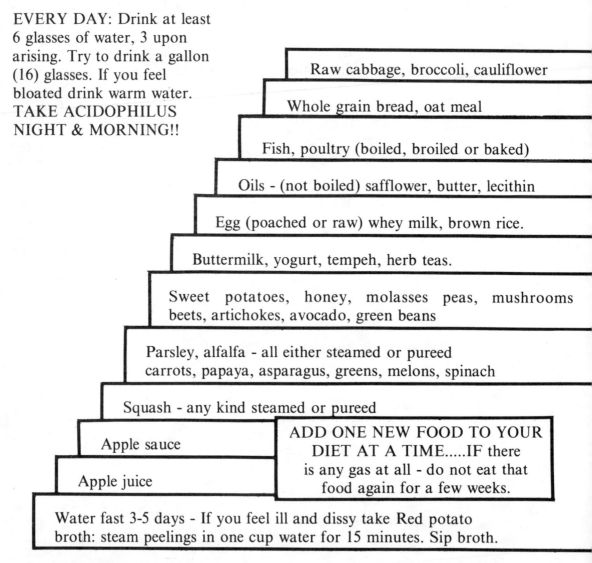

Raw cabbage, broccoli, cauliflower

Whole grain bread, oat meal

Fish, poultry (boiled, broiled or baked)

Oils - (not boiled) safflower, butter, lecithin

Egg (poached or raw) whey milk, brown rice.

Buttermilk, yogurt, tempeh, herb teas.

Sweet potatoes, honey, molasses peas, mushrooms beets, artichokes, avocado, green beans

Parsley, alfalfa - all either steamed or pureed carrots, papaya, asparagus, greens, melons, spinach

Squash - any kind steamed or pureed

Apple sauce

ADD ONE NEW FOOD TO YOUR DIET AT A TIME.....IF there is any gas at all - do not eat that food again for a few weeks.

Apple juice

Water fast 3-5 days - If you feel ill and dissy take Red potato broth: steam peelings in one cup water for 15 minutes. Sip broth.

EAT SIMPLY — preferably only one food at a time, two at the most.

ABSOLUTELY DO NOT EAT OR CONSUME:
Cheese, nuts, peanuts, alcohol, tobacco, ground meat, meat loaves, white flour, sugar (white or brown), salt, coffee, tea, shortnings, pop, cola, kool aid type drinks, breakfast type drinks, candies, cookies, cakes, pies, ice cream, or street drugs. If you must take medication double or triple your acidophilus intake.

Any questions call Patti at 763-4436

GOOD HEALTH TO YOU.

CORRECT FOOD COMBINATIONS

Monotrophic Diet--One food at a Meal is Ideal.

DO NOT EAT: Proteins with Starches, or Protein with Fruit,
except: Avocado and Coconuts combine well with *Acid* and
Sub-acid fruits. Seeds and Nuts combine well with *Acid* fruits.

DO NOT EAT: Any kind of fruit with starch, *Acid* and
Sweet fruits together, fruits and vegetables together, or any more
than 4 foods from either *Fruits* or *Vegetables* at a meal.

DO EAT:

Melons alone.
Only one *Protein* or one *Starch* at a meal.

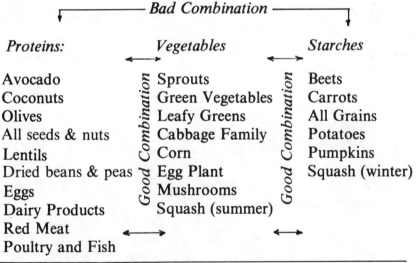

FOOD BEST FOR HUMAN CONSUMPTION

Best

Bean Sprouts
Bran
Wheat germ
Oats
Garlic
Brown Rice
Low-fat fish
Dark green leafy Vegetables
Sweet Potatoes

Fair

Peanut Butter
Cream
Most Cheeses
Whole Milk
Fatty Fish
Butter
Pizza
Salad Oils
Avocado
Less-fatty Beef and Lamb
Eggs
Canned Juices and Vegetables
Cottage Cheese
Dried Fruits
Granola
Ice Cream
Veal
Whole Milk Yogurt
Margarine
Deep-fried Poultry
or Fish

Good

Whole Grain Goods
Nuts
Most Fresh Fruits and Vegetables
White Potatoes
Herb Teas
Beans (legumes)
Skim Milk
Poultry (without the skin)
Sunflower seeds
Low-fat Yogurt
Unsalted Vegetable juices
Tempeh
Buttermilk
Unsweetened Fruit Juices

Least Desirable

Potato Chips
Soda Pop
Sausage
Pretzels
Coffee
Pie
Pickles
Chocolate
Salted Snacks
Soup mixes
Coffee whitener
White Flour
Olives
Sugar
Lard
Tea
Salt
Port
Cake
French Fries
Fatty Meats

HYPOGLYCEMIA DIET

HYPOGLYEMIA DIET (see section on Special Diets and Recipes)

Upon arising: Medium orange, half grapefruit, or 4 oz. of fresh juice.

BREAKFAST: Fruit or 4 oz. of fresh juice; 1 egg with or without Protein Powder; ONLY ONE slice of PATTI'S BREAD or toast with plenty of butter; Herbal Beverage.

2 hours later: 4 oz. fresh juice.

LUNCH: Meat, fish, cheese or eggs: salad (large serving of raw vegetables); ONLY ONE slice of PATTI'S BREAD with butter; Herbal Tea.

3 hours later: 8 oz. of milk or buttermilk

**1 hour before
  dinner:** 4 oz. of fresh juice.

DINNER: Soup; Vegetables (Steamed or raw) liberal portion of meat, fish or poultry; ONLY ONE slice of PATTI'S BREAD; Herbal Beverage or Herbal Tea.

**Every 2 hours
  until bed:** 4 oz. milk, buttermilk or a small handful of nuts.

Allowable Vegetables:

Asparagus, avocado, beets, broccoli, brussel sprouts, cabbage, cauliflower, carrots, celery, corn, cucumbers, eggplant, lima beans, onions, peas, radishes, sauerkraut, squash, stringbeans, tomatoes, turnips, greens.

Allowable Fruits:

Apples, apricots, berries, grapefruit, melons, oranges, peaches, pears, pineapple, tangerines.

May be cooked or raw, with or without cream, but without sugar; canned fruits should be packed in water, not syrup. The raw are better if enjoyed that way.

Allowable Protein:

Protein Powder, poultry, fish, dairy products, mushrooms, eggs. Vegetable protein.

Allowable Juices:

Any unsweetened fruit or vegetable juice.

Allowable Beverages:

Herbal Beverage, Herbal Teas.

Avoid Absolutely:

Alcoholic and soft drinks, sugar, candy and other sweets, Caffein, Potatoes, rice, grapes, raisins, plums, figs, dates, bananas, spaghetti, macaroni, noodles, doughnuts, jams, jellies, marmalades.

PATTI BREAD

Combine:
- 1/2 C. Oils
- 2 C. Hot Water
- 2 t. Sea Salt
- 1/4 to 1/3 C. Black Strap Molasses

Combine and heat until yeast grows to 1 Cup.
- 1/2 C. warm water
- 1 Envelope Dried Yeast
- 1 T. Brown Sugar

Beat:
- 2 Eggs

Combine:
- 3 C. Whole Wheat Flour
- 4½ C. Unbleached Flour
- 1/2 C. Protein Powder

Mix all ingredients together. Let raise until volume doubles (1½ hours) Knead. Separate into 4 loaves. Knead. Oil tops of loaves. Let raise until volume doubles (1½ hours) Bake 35-45 minutes at 350 degrees.

POTASSIUM BROTH

Celery Tops and Leaves
Sliced Onions
Carrot Tops
Red Potato Peels
Green Beans
   Simmer for 1 hour, then strain or blend in blender.

SECTION THREE
CLEANSES AND ENEMAS

SEVEN DAY CLEANSE

Day before starting cleanse eat only fruits and vegetables. Night before 2 capsules of Cascara Sagrada. Eat nothing (other than specified) for seven days. Drink plenty of pure water (5 glasses additional). You may have herbal teas, herbal beverages, vegetable broths or juice.

You will need these items:
> 16 ounce glass or jar.
> Juice (your choice of Apple, Berry, Pineapple, Grape, or Herbal Punch).
> Enema Bag.
> Ground coffee.
> Garlic capsules (opened).
> 2 quart bottles of Hydrated Bentonite.
> 12 ounces of Powdered Psyllium Hulls.
> 1 pint liquid Chlorophyll.
> Fasting Herbs: licorice, Hawthorn, Beet Powder, Fennel.
> Natural vitamin and mineral supplement — 70 capsules.
> Calcium — 70 capsules.
> Chewable C — 70 tablets.
> Cascara Sagrada.

Directions:
> 5 times/day, every 3 hours do the following
>> Pour 4 ounces juice into 16 ounce glass or jar.
>> Add 8 ounces pure water
>> Add 1 T. Liquid Chlorophyll
>> Add 4 T. Bentonite
>> Add 1 T. Psyllium Hulls
>> Stir well. Drink immediately. Follow with additional glass of pure water.

> 5 times/day — 1½ hours after drinking the above, take the following:
>> 2 Vitamin and mineral supplements
>> 2 Calcium
>> 2 Fasting Herbs
>> 2 Cascara Sagrada or as many as necessary to have several bowel movements/day.

Enema

It is of utmost importance to take a daily enema while on this cleanse. Either Coffee or Garlic Enemas (See Enemas).

Next Week

Take Acidophilus the last thing at night and the first thing in the morning. Very important to build back bacteria in your colon.

EYE WASH

1 Capsule (broken) Herbal Eye Wash (Golden Seal, Bayberry, Eyebright, Red Raspberry Leaves, Capsicum—optional)
1 Cup pure water, boiled. Let steep for 20 minutes. Strain through cotton balls in bottom of funnel or tea strainer. Use eye cup or eye dropper. Blind the eye a few times. Let eye rest. Repeat. The eye may sting; if unbearable use more water. Use eye wash at least 3 times a day. TRY to keep eye opened while dropping eye wash in. Keep using less and less water as you can stand it. Make new solution every 2 days. NEVER use same eyewash portion twice; use fresh solution with each eye.

ENEMAS (See section on CLEANSING)
ENEMAS

When the colon is congested, toxins are absorbed back into the system, manifesting themselves as fever, earache, sore throat, headache, or other illness.

Capsicum — 1/2 teasp. to bag of pure water.

Garlic - Blend 1 or 2 garlic buds for each bag in 1 quart water. Strain. Add enough water to fill bag. Do 3 times.

Catnip — 2 Tsp. catnip (18 capsules) in 1 quart water. Strain, Add enough water to fill bag.

Mineral Water — 1/2 cup to bag of water.

Slippery Elm — 1 Tbsp. powder (9 capsules) in blender with 1 pint pure water. Add enough water to fill the bag.

White Oak Bark — 2 Tbsp. powder (18 capsules) in blender with 1 pint water (pure). Then bring to a boil, steep for 20 min. Add enough water to fill bag.

Coffee — 1 cup strong brewed coffee (not instant or decafinated). Add enough water to fill bag.

Directions

Place long enema tube or douche tube up rectum while lying on left side. Control water by the valve so water enter comfortable. Keep water for up to 10 minutes then expel. Refill bag, go through the above steps, then slowly turn on your back. Keep water for up to 10 minutes, then expel. Refill bag, go through the above steps then slowly turn to your right side. keep water for up to 10 minutes then expel.

Always take acidophilus, yogurt, buttermilk or kefir to replace the natural bacteria in the colon after taking enemas.

SECTION FOUR
LYMPHATIC SYSTEM

1	Hypothalmus	26	Liver
2	Anterior Pituitary	27	Stomach
3	Posterior Pituitary	28	Stomach Hydrochloric Acid
4	Pineal	29	Pancreas Blood Sugar
5	Ear	30	Pancreas Enzymes
6	Eye	31	Cardiac Valves
7	Nose	32	Solar Plexus
8	Teeth	33	Spleen
9	Gums	34	Gall Bladder
10	Parotid	35	Transverse Colon
11	Sublingual Lymph	36	Ascending Colon
12	Tonsils	37	Descending Colon
13	Adenoids	38	Sigmoid Colon
14	Carotid Sinus	39	Ileocecal Valve
15	Hair	40	Appendix
16	Parathyroid	41	Pyloic Valve
17	Thyroid	42	Small Intestines
18	Lung	43	Uterus or Prostate
19	Thymus	45	Ovaries or Testes
20	Bronchial	46	Kidney
21	Lymph	47	Adrenal Medulla
22	Diaphragm	48	Adrenal Cortex
23	Heart	49	Femoral Lymph
24	Breast Lymph	50	Skin
25	Breast Milk Ducts	51	Bones

GLAND CHART

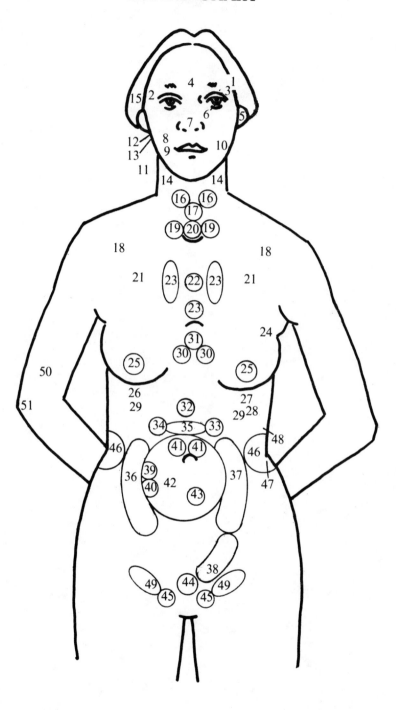

LYMPHATIC SYSTEM

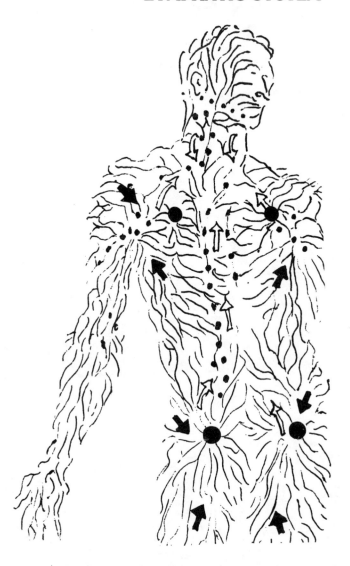

Lymph is an absorbent substance capable of collecting 3 waste products generated by the cells of the body, and turning them over to the blood. The blood, in turn, transports the wastes to the lungs, kidneys, colon, and skin for elimination from the body.

The pervasive lymphatic system which returns fluids from tissue spaces to the circulation is something like a bailing mechanism that keeps a boat from floundering. *Lymph* is collected from small vessels that merge into large ones (black arrows) and is returned (white arrows) to the right side of the heart through veins in the area of the neck. *Lymph Nodes* along the course of the lymphatic vessels act as filter-traps of bacteria to arrest the spread of infections.

BIBLIOGRAPHY

The American People's Encyclopedia. Vol. I, pp 943-946.

Awake, Brooklyn, New York, Watchtower Bible and Tract Society. July 22, 1978 and December 22, 1980.

Barton, John and Margaret. *Emotions Can Heal,* U.S.A. John E. Barton, 1980.

Carter, Albert E. *The Miracles of Rebound Exercise.* U.S.A. Snohomish Publishing Co., Inc., 1979.

Chan, Pedzr. *Finger Acupressure.* U.S.A. Ballantine Books, 1975.

Chang, Stephen T. *The Book of Internal Exercises.* U.S.A. Strawberry Hill Press, 1978.

Christopher, John R. *School of Natural Healing.* Provo, Utah: Microlith Printing, 1976.

Cooley, Donald G. *Family Medical Guide.* New York: Meredith Corp. 1964.

Dale, Ralph Alan, *Acupuncture with your Fingers.* "Alternatives" December 1978, pp. 22-35.

Healthview Newsletter. Vol. 10. Charlottesville, Va.

Herbalist. Vol. 1 #1. p. 34, 1976.

Ritchason, Jack. *The Little Herb Encyclopedia* and *The Little Vitamin and Mineral Encyclopedia.* U.S.A. Thornwood Books, 1980.

Royal, Penny C. *Herbally Yours.* Provo, Utah: BiWorld Publishers Inc., 1979.

Weiss, Jennifer and Burnett, Vena. *Colon Cleanse the Easy Way!* (Pamphlet)

West, Samuel T. *The Lymphatic Exercise Home-Study Program.* (Pamphlet)

About the Author:

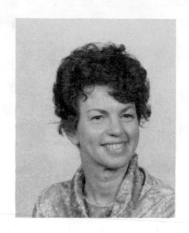

PATTI C. LLOYD is a graduate of Michigan State University in Foods and Nutrition, and has taught in the United States and Europe. She is a licensed cosmetologist in Michigan, Missouri and California, and has owned her own Health and Beauty Salon where most of the research was done for her book, "ACU-ENERGY". She is working presently with her husband as a Nutritional Consultant and Herbalist.

ISBN-0-89557-060-2